Computers in Health Care

Kathryn J. Hannah   Marion J. Ball
Series Editors

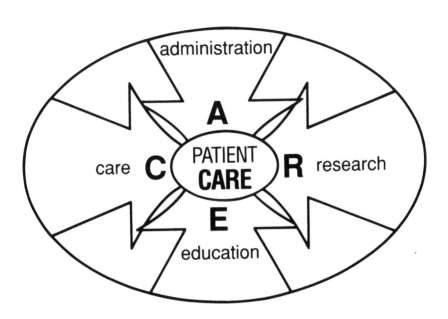

Springer

New York
Berlin
Heidelberg
Barcelona
Budapest
Hong Kong
London
Milan
Paris
Santa Clara
Singapore
Tokyo

Computers in Health Care

Series Editors:
Kathryn J. Hannah   Marion J. Ball

Kimball I. Maull
Jeffrey S. Augenstein
Editors

Trauma Informatics

With a Foreword by Donald D. Trunkey

With 55 Illustrations

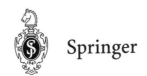 Springer

Kimball I. Maull, MD, FACS
Professor and Vice Chairman
Department of Surgery
Stritch School of Medicine
Director, Division of Trauma and
  Emergency Medical Services
Loyola University Medical Center
Maywood, IL 60153
USA

Jeffrey S. Augenstein, MD, PhD, FACS
Professor
Departments of Surgery and
  Anesthesiology
Director, Computer Services
Ryder Trauma Center
University of Miami School of Medicine
Miami, FL 33136
USA

Cover photo © Ed Kashi/PHOTOTAKE NYC

Library of Congress Cataloging-in-Publication Data
Trauma informatics / [edited by] Kimball I. Maull, Jeffrey S. Augenstein,
    p. cm. — (Computers and health care)
  Includes index.
  ISBN 0-387-94359-5 (hardcover : alk paper)
  1. Traumatology.   2. Medical informatics.   3. Trauma centers—Data
processing.   I. Maull, Kimball I. (Kimball Ivan), 1942–   .
II. Augenstein, Jeffrey S.   III. Series.
  [DNLM: 1. Wounds and Injuries.   2. Medical Informatics.
3. Registries.   WO 700 T77566   1997]
  RD93.T688   1997
  617.1′00285—dc21
  DNLM/DLC
  for Library of Congress   97-8491

Printed on acid-free paper.

Production coordinated by Chernow Editorial Services, Inc., and managed by Bill Imbornoni;
manufacturing supervised by Jeffrey Taub.
Typeset by Best-set Typesetter Ltd., Hong Kong.
Printed and bound by Maple-Vail Book Manufacturing Group, York, PA.
Printed in the United States of America.

9 8 7 6 5 4 3 2 1

ISBN 0-387-94359-5 Springer-Verlag New York Berlin Heidelberg   SPIN 10476075

Foreword

Information and the technology to rapidly transmit, analyze, document, and disperse this information are increasing arithmetically, if not logarithmically. Arguably, no discipline better exemplifies this trend than medicine. It can be further argued that care of the trauma patient is one of the better examples of informatics and the potential benefit to the health professionals who care for these patients. Maull and Augenstein have provided us with a primer on informatics and its use in trauma care. The subject matter is timely and covers the gamut of trauma care from prehospital to rehabilitation.

Who will benefit from trauma informatics? A simple answer would be anyone who takes care of trauma patients. From a broader perspective, however, at least three examples illustrate how trauma informatics can be used today to exert a positive effect on patient outcome. The first example is care of combat casualties, including battlefield resuscitation, evacuation, acute care, and ultimate return to the continental United States. Current technology is such that via global positioning satellite, a corpsman could transmit to a remote area the vital signs and pertinent physical findings of a combat casualty. Furthermore, the location of the corpsman and the casualty would be precisely known, and consultation and destination disposition would be possible. The injured person, when admitted to a combat support hospital, could be continuously monitored and additional remote consultation obtained. Subsequent care and evacuation to an appropriate facility out of the combat region or back to the United States would continue to rely on the tracking system and consultation capability.

It has been said that good judgment comes from experience. Unfortunately, experience comes from bad judgment. From this aphorism it is readily appreciated that consultation with an experienced trauma surgeon may be advantageous for patient outcome. Thus, physicians who only occasionally see and treat trauma patients could, through informatics, have direct consultation with more experienced surgeons who see and treat trauma patients on a regular basis. X-ray films could be put into digital format and transmitted with the request for diagnostic consultation. Operative decisions and management of the patient in the intensive care setting could be made jointly. Transfers would be made easier with direct consultation with the receiving hospital from the health care providers in the transport vehicle.

Examples of the future use of trauma informatics are provided by such projects as Space Station Freedom and subsequent extraterrestrial NASA endeavors. Health care providers on the space platform can have direct consultation with a number of centers for trauma expertise.

The examples—providing care of combat casualties, as well as opportunities for consultation in present practice and in space—serve to highlight the potential utility of *Trauma Informatics*. However, the applications of trauma informatics are limited only by our imagination. I recommend this book as a place to start and to provoke us to redefine what is possible in information sharing and decision making.

Donald D. Trunkey

Series Preface

This series is intended for the rapidly increasing number of health care professionals who have rudimentary knowledge and experience in health care computing and are seeking opportunities to expand their horizons. It does not attempt to compete with the primers already on the market. Eminent international experts will edit, author, or contribute to each volume in order to provide comprehensive and current accounts of innovations and future trends in this quickly evolving field. Each book will be practical, easy to use, and well referenced.

Our aim is for the series to encompass all of the health professions by focusing on specific professions, such as nursing, in individual volumes. However, integrated computing systems are only one tool for improving communication among members of the health care team. Therefore, it is our hope that the series will stimulate professionals to explore additional means of fostering interdisciplinary exchanges.

This series springs from a professional collaboration that has grown over the years into a highly valued personal friendship. Our joint values put people first. If the Computers in Health Care series lets us share those values by helping health care professionals to communicate their ideas for the benefit of patients, then our efforts will have succeeded.

Kathryn J. Hannah
Marion J. Ball

Preface

In 1978 R Adams Cowley, a leading pioneer in improving care of the injured, engineered a disaster exercise at the Friendship Airport (currently Baltimore Washington International) in Baltimore, mimicking an airplane crash with moulaged victims and a regional EMS response. Using an unwieldy video camera and a satellite transmitter (COMSAT) that took up the space of half a flatbed truck, Dr. Cowley sent real-time images of burned victims to experts standing by at the Brooke Army Medical Center's burn unit in San Antonio, Texas, thus demonstrating that an accurate determination of depth and degree of burn injury could be made from halfway across the country. In 1997 at the International Conference on Communication and Electronic Innovations in Emergency Care in Regensburg, Germany, Dr. H. Reichle, director of the Insitute for Air Medicine, demonstrated an actual trauma patient in Pilsen, Czech Republic, on the screen of a personal computer and held discussions with the attending surgeon regarding the need for and means of transporting the patient to a higher level of trauma care. Using technology comparatively rudimentary by today's standards, Dr. Cowley convinced others of his vision of the future almost 20 years ago. Today, linking the computer and the video camera has opened new horizons for simultaneous consultation and timely decision making that directly affect patient outcome. Indeed, technologically speaking, those who earlier this decade professed that the sky was the limit were clearly short-sighted!

In *Trauma Informatics* the editors have attempted to redefine trauma care, not in a futuristic sense, but by portraying the potential impact of existing technological advances on how we assess, resuscitate, and manage patients with significant injuries. Common to what we do as trauma care providers is the art and science of communication. The language of communication is documentation. Without documentation, we cannot learn from what we have done right nor from what we have done wrong. If our own errors or the mistakes of others are not documented, we are condemned to repeat them, much to the patient's (and our own!) disadvantage. An additional caveat is that communication must be rapid and accurate. In the trauma setting, so often the provider must make lifesaving decisions quickly, under highly adverse circumstances, and with an incomplete database. The challenge for informatics in trauma care is to be able to respond rapidly and factually, and to adjust in real time to the ever changing demands of the clinical setting.

In the opening chapter, the editors provide a glimpse of the role of finely tuned and coordinated informatics on a hypothetical injured patient and proceed to prove that there is little difference between the hypothetical and the real. One of the editors (JA) describes the actual workings of one of the country's most advanced trauma centers and the role of informatics in resuscitation, continuing care, and research involving the critically injured.

Section II includes the role of informatics in optimizing prehospital trauma care, examining the use of computerized ambulance run sheets organized for user-friendly application and the improved opportunities for meaningful quality improvement and monitoring. The chapter on vehicle crash investigation introduces the language of biomechanics into the equation and serves by example and description to emphasize mechanism of injury in the orderly assessment of the victim of road-related trauma. These two chapters come together in the chapter on emergency department (ED) informatics, which provides important concepts for documentation and sources for additional customized systems, which may be tailored to the needs of the reader. The chapter on emergency radiology adds to our knowledge of how radiologic advances have changed our clinical practice and our practical approach to the injured. A look at the role of informatics in the intensive care unit truly distills much of what is potentially beneficial for patient care into what is actually achievable in a state of the art unit. The authors critically evaluate the role of informatics in the everyday setting of a busy ICU and convincingly present data on how interventions can be better documented, costs reduced, and care improved. A comprehensive look at rehabilitation and the need for accurate and reproducible data completes Section II. In this highly informative chapter, the experts leave little doubt that an organized approach to rehabilitation is worth the investment but add a note of caution that, perhaps more than at any other phase in trauma care, informatics is crucial for documentation.

Section III concentrates on trauma registries and emphasizes the critical need for accuracy in data acquisition and transmission. The initial chapter provides the groundwork for the organizational and functional aspects of reliable registries. The subsequent chapters provide a more focused look at trauma registries, which begin, in all circumstances, in the hospital. This material provides a foundation for discussions of how these data are used at the state level and, finally, to reach a national database. The authors identify both the potential benefits and the pitfalls of registry informatics and underscore the power of a large data set in establishing standards of care.

Section IV completes the work with a most important submission on the role of trauma informatics in establishing, monitoring, and maturing clinical pathways/guidelines for care of specific injuries, critical care interventions, and quality improvement. From the perspective of cost effectiveness while maintaining quality of patient care, the principles embodied in this chapter comprise a suitable ending to this work.

The editors express their profound thanks to the editorial staff at Springer-Verlag for patience and vision in seeing this project to completion. Special thanks is due to Kelley Suttenfield for her gentle but firm reminders that the value of this book can be realized only if it is published (!) and to Bill Day for his continued support.

Kimball I. Maull
Jeffrey S. Augenstein

Contents

SECTION III

SECTION IV

Contributors

Jeffrey S. Augenstein, MD, PhD, FACS
Professor, Departments of Surgery and Anesthesiology, Director, Computer Services, Ryder Trauma Center, University of Miami School of Medicine, Miami, FL, USA

Wayne S. Copes, PhD
Vice President, Tri-Analytics, Inc., Bel Air, MD, USA

Linda C. Degutis, DrPH
Assistant Professor, Department of Surgery, Co-Director, Regional Injury Prevention Program, Yale University, New Haven, USA

Thomas J. Esposito, MD, MPH, FACS
Associate Professor, Department of Surgery, Assistant Director for Injury Analysis and Prevention Programs, Loyola University Burn and Shock Trauma Institute, Loyola University Medical Center, Maywood, IL, USA

Michael E. Flisak, MD
Associate Professor and Vice Chairman, Department of Radiology, Loyola University Medical Center, Maywood, IL, USA

Carl P. Granger, MD
Director, Center for Functional Assessment Research, School of Medicine and Biomedical Sciences, State University of New York, Buffalo, NY, USA

Jeffrey S. Hecht, MD
Associate Professor, Departments of Medicine and Surgery, University of Tennessee Graduate School of Medicine, Director, Patricia Neal Rehabilitation Center, Knoxville, TN, USA

Mark C. Henry, MD, FACEP
Professor and Chairman, Department of Emergency Medicine, State University of New York, Stony Brook, NY, USA

Lester Kallus, MD
Assistant Clinical Professor, Department of Emergency Medicine, State University of New York, Stony Brook, NY, USA

Alfred G. Kaye, MS, CTRS
Manager, Recreation Therapy and Quality Improvement, Patricia Neal Rehabilitation Institute, Knoxville, TN, USA

M. Jack Lee, MS, EMT-P
Director of Information Services, Albuquerque Ambulance Service, Albuquerque, NM, USA

G. Daniel Martich, MD
Assistant Professor, Department of Anesthesiology and Critical Care Medicine, University of Pittsburgh School of Medicine, Pittsburgh, PA, USA

Anthony J. Martinez, EMT-P
Director, Quality Improvement, Albuquerque Ambulance Service, Albuquerque, NM, USA

Kimball I. Maull, MD, FACS
Professor and Vice Chairman, Department of Surgery, Director, Division of Trauma and Emergency Medical Services, Loyola University Medical Center, Maywood, IL, USA

Dietmar Otte, PhD
Director, Accident Research Unit, Medical University Hannover, Hannover, Germany

Michael D. Pasquale, MD
Attending Traumatologist, Lehigh Valley Hospital Center, Allentown, PA, USA

Andrew B. Peitzman, MD
Professor, Department of Surgery, University of Pittsburgh School of Medicine, Pittsburgh, PA, USA

Gregory D. Powell, MD
Assistant Professor, Department of Rehabilitation Medicine, University of Texas Health Sciences Center, San Antonio, TX, USA

Michael Rhodes, MD, FACS
Professor, Department of Surgery, Jefferson Medical School, Chairman, Department of Surgery, Medical Center of Delaware, Wilmington, DE, USA

Charles L. Rice, MD, FACS
Professor and Vice Dean, Department of Surgery, University of Illinois School of Medicine, Chicago, IL, USA

Leticia M. Rutledge, BA
Trauma Registrar, State of New Mexico, Albuquerque, NM, USA

Robert Rutledge, MD, FACS
Associate Professor of Surgery, University of North Carolina, Chapel Hill, NC, USA

William J. Sacco, PhD
President, Tri-Analytics, Inc., Bel Air, MD, USA

Carl A. Sirio, MD
Assistant Professor, Department of Anesthesiology and Critical Care Medicine, University of Pittsburgh School of Medicine, Pittsburgh, PA, USA

Todd B. Taylor, MD, FACEP
Attending Physician, Department of Emergency Medicine, Good Samaritan Regional Medical Center, Phoenix Children's Hospital, Phoenix, AZ, USA

Donald D. Trunkey, MD, FACS
Professor and Chairman, Department of Surgery, Oregon Health Sciences University School of Medicine, Portland, OR, USA

Peter Viccellio, MD, FACEP
Associate Professor and Vice Chairman, Department of Emergency Medicine, State University of New York, Stony Brook, NY, USA

Sheryl Zougras, RN, BSN
Trauma Registrar, Loyola University Medical Center, Coordinator, Trauma Information Systems, Loyola University Burn & Shock Trauma Institute, Maywood, IL, USA

Section I

1
Trauma Informatics: Today's Vision, Tomorrow's Concepts

JEFFREY S. AUGENSTEIN AND KIMBALL I. MAULL

One night in the not-too-distant future, a driver falls asleep at the wheel on an isolated highway, and his car crashes into a tree. Fortunately, the car is equipped with a crash-sensing system, which immediately begins a lifesaving process. First, the system automatically calls 911 and provides the coordinates of the crash, as received from GPS, the satellite-based global positioning system. A voice enunciator asks the driver to speak to the operator if he can. But since the driver is unable to respond, the system transmits information on the crash characteristics, including the vehicle's instantaneous change in velocity.

After receiving the call, the 911 operator dispatches emergency medical services (EMS) personnel and police to the crash location. Because the driver did not respond and the crash force was severe, the emergency team assumes that the driver is critically injured and dispatches a helicopter to transport him to the nearest Level 1 trauma center, saving important time.

Upon arrival at the crash scene, the rescue team find the driver's "smart card," which contains a microprocessor and data file covering his entire health history. When the card is inserted into a terminal on the helicopter, it discloses that the driver has a history of mitral valve disease with treatment including Coumadin. As a part of the advanced life support (ALS) activities, the EMS crew attaches the patient to a physiological monitor that transmits data on heart rate, blood pressure, and oxygen saturation to physicians 25 miles away at the trauma center. Meanwhile, the police and EMS personnel fill out electronic forms on the crash, and document the scene with a portable camera that sends digital pictures of the car and the injured driver to the trauma center.

Computerized data have been flowing into the electronic record at the trauma center from the moment the 911 call was received. By the time the patient arrives, all the prehospital data and past medical history are already in the trauma center's computer system. A nationwide clinical database is accessed to obtain information not contained in the patient's smart card.

In the trauma room, physiological monitoring is done continuously by the center's equipment. The admitting physician enters her notes and orders on the trauma room's workstation, using a menu-based system for diagnostic and procedure descriptions. When free-form text is required to illuminate a point, the clinician types in the information, or dictates it into the computer's voice transcription system. The patient's injuries are shown graphically via diagrams generated by the system from information entered by the clinician.

Because all images including x-rays, scans, photographs, and diagrams are stored in digital form, physicians using workstations throughout the trauma center are able to review and evaluate the patient's injuries. The surgeon in the operating room could review a brain CAT scan at the same time the radiologist is discussing it with a colleague. If necessary, the digitized x-ray films could be transmitted to an expert at a distant hospital via a nationwide high speed network.

Very little of the data in the flowsheet section of the patient's medical record was entered by hand. Physiological measurements, ventilator parameters, infusion rates, and output quantities were all obtained electronically. To indicate when medications were administrated, a nurse scanned drug containers with a bar-code reader. After the physician entered orders into the system and the nurse acknowledged them, the system created or updated the Kardex. In fact, nurses were notified by bedside workstations when activities were due. This integrated approach to medical record keeping allows the attending physician to make associations within the data, such as checking for any contradictions with respect to when a medication order was entered. The interactive system also greatly facilitated the trauma center's utilization review effort.

Thanks in part to the rapid flow of electronic information, the trauma center staff was able to save this patient's life. In addition, the information system allowed the trauma center to receive complete insurance information and rapidly generate an accurate bill for services. The menu-based diagnostic and procedure description system allowed clinicians to summarize the patient's complex injuries and treatments quickly and completely. The system then translated its internal language, the Structured Nomenclature of Medicine (SNOMED), into required terms, such as the International Classification of Diseases (ICD), Current Procedural Terminology (CPT), and the Abbreviated Injury Scale (AIS). Information on this case was transmitted to a national trauma registry and other research databases, assisting ongoing efforts to improve quality of care and reduce service costs.

Many of the technologies described in this scenario of the future are in daily use or may be encountered in some real-world evaluations. Even the crash-notification-enabled automobile is available today. General Motors markets Cadillacs equipped with GPS links and cellular telephones that will call an 800 number, confirming that the vehicle has crashed. The National

Highway Traffic Safety Administration is funding a project in Buffalo, New York, where researchers are placing a transducer module capable of defining the crash conditions in addition to a GPS equipment and a cellular telephone in one thousand automobiles. These cars not only will be capable of expressing that they have crashed, they also will be able to communicate the magnitude and direction of the crash forces. Clearly these new technologies may improve the response time of emergency services to crash victims, particularly in isolated environments. Information about the crash may optimize the trauma center's care by enabling clinicians to apply biomechanical principles to patient management. Injury patterns may be anticipated and those insights applied to the patient evaluation.

The remaining parts of the scenario are, as previously stated, present to some degree in many hospitals. The Ryder Trauma Center at the University of Miami Jackson Memorial Medical Center in Miami, Florida, contains many of the scenario's information system components. The center, which opened in the spring of 1992, was designed as an information-enabled building. This chapter summarizes the structure of the internally developed CARE Information System and the strategies underlying it.

Ryder Trauma Center

The CARE Information System: Description

The Ryder Trauma Center encompasses over 138,000 ft² within its four floors and basement. At the top, a helipad provides access to even large military aircraft. Two elevators, each able to hold a pair of patient, as well as clinicians, supporting and equipment, can make the journey to the first floor within 15 seconds. The first floor level houses 5 resuscitation bays, a 6-bed observation unit, 6 operating rooms, a 10-bed postanesthetic recovery unit, a family waiting room, a conference/press room, an angiographic suite, a helical CAT scan, and two stationary x-ray suites. The second floor holds a 20-bed intensive care unit, additional family waiting rooms, classrooms, physician and staff offices, a raised-floor computer room, and a communications equipment room. The two information system support rooms and their respective air conditioning systems are supplied by the hospital's uninterruptible power. In-room power conditioning shields the electronics from power fluctuations, particularly during switches to emergency power. Each clinical area on the first and second floors is equipped to support an intensive care level of monitoring and intervention. The third floor houses 60 routine-care beds. The fourth floor contains a 55-bed brain injury and orthopedic injury rehabilitation unit.

An Ethernet network, with presently 300 access points, supports connections at each point of care (e.g., operating room) and each administrative and educational location (e.g., secretarial desktop). A star configuration is used, with all connections terminating in hubs in the communications equipment room.

The acronym CARE refers to the clinical, administrative, research, and educational functionality of the computer system in place at the Ryder Trauma Center. The underlying concept is that the latter three functions can be facilitated through a clinical information management system. The administrative and research functions in a trauma center are largely fed from clinical information.

The administrative functions include hospital and professional billing, quality assurance reporting, and utilization review assessment. Typically separate teams individually perform each of these functions; the initial step is review of the medical record. This often creates competition for the paper chart among workers from these groups as well as the clinicians who are responsible for the patient.

Professional billing is generated by the different clinicians who simultaneously participate in the patient's care. For a trauma patient this may include the general surgeon, specialty surgeons such as orthopedic and neurological surgeons, anesthesiologists, radiologists, pathologists who interpret laboratory and anatomic specimens, psychiatrists, intensivists, and other nonsurgical specialists. Many personnel resources are expended on this function. Heretofore various departmental billing personnel often did not communicate or coordinate activities. It is possible that the same patient with one set of problems could be described differently by various professional/billing strategies. These approaches may conflict with the hospital's billing descriptions.

The duplication of effort and the potential for incorrect and uncoordinated billing can be obviated if the clinicians assign problem description terminology as a part of their respective note writing. Billing codes can then be created directly from these precise clinical descriptions. This is being done in the CARE system. As a part of the care delivery process, the various treating physicians, nurses, and technicians develop a precise clinical problem list.

The quality assurance effort in trauma centers is mandated by local, state, and federal governments as well as regulatory bodies such as the Joint Commission on the Accreditation of Health care Organizations (JCAHO). Numerous reports, in a series that addresses basic registry information through quality of care analyses, are required, often on a monthly basis. The traditional approach involves individuals who review charts as well as analyze primary reports (e.g., weekly morbidity and mortality conference summaries). It is central to the CARE system concept that much of the required data can be created by clinicians in the process of care. If documents (e.g., operative records) are created as computerized forms, much of the required quality assurance data elements can be made available. These data include times at which diagnostic or therapeutic interventions commenced and patient status information such as systematic blood pressure at these various times. If the responsible physicians and nurses are the primary source of the data, there appear to be low error rates; personnel whose sole responsibility is quality assurance can be kept to a minimum.

In the CARE system, data required for quality assurance are automatically transferred into the quality assurance database. The CARE system software looks for completeness of the individual patient records as well as for internal consistencies. For example, a patient designated as sustaining trauma during pregnancy should be female, and the system checks to determine whether the patient is described appropriately. If the pregnant patient is not listed as female in the "sex" field, the system includes the patient in an exceptions report. Personnel can then address these inconsistencies.

Education is an integral component of a trauma center's function. Staff includes attending level physicians, physicians in training, medical and nursing students, nurses, technicians such as respiratory and radiology technicians, and administrative personnel. Computer systems can augment the dissemination of knowledge and the evaluation of individual clinicians' knowledge.

The CARE system supports the discrimination of information in a number of ways. The first is the provision of multimedia-based lectures. Computer workstations can provide an interactive type of videotaped lecture. Inexpensive video cameras allow clinicians to capture images of injuries and complex procedures such as abdominal operations. These films then provide a ready source of materials that can be digitized and included in multimedia presentations. The ability to digitize voice allows narrative to easily be included in presentations.

The other strategy for information dissemination provided by the CARE system is the provision of reference materials. A number of functions are available at all workstations, including access to all policies and procedures of the Ryder Trauma Center and to hospital charge lists. The personal computer workstations distributed throughout the Ryder Trauma Center provide access to these sources of information as well as to the database MEDLINE.

A multiple-choice examination function can be provided at each workstation. Tests are available in many subjects and can coordinate difficulty to level of the examinee's training. Clinicians are provided instantaneous feedback on their performance.

Additional sources of information provided by the CARE system are electronic mail, a bulletin board of scheduled events, and a telephone directory. The policy and procedure manual is available through the electronic mail system. It is often critical that affected staff be informed when relevant policies or procedures change or are added or deleted. When a clinical supervisor changes a policy or procedure, electronic mail is immediately sent to the ED parties affected. In addition, the supervisor is provided with a report indicating which clinicians have read the messages. Quality assurance reviews often evaluate the method for confirming that staff has been informed about policy or procedure changes. Managing this information in a manual system can be extremely labor intensive.

The clinical functionality of the CARE system is its most complex aspect. It provides the ability to enter and review components of the medical record throughout the Ryder Trauma Center. Data are acquired through each clinician's entry and from other computers via electronic exchange. The following systems provide data to the CARE system.

The Jackson Memorial Hospital information system provides admission, discharge, and transfer data; as well as laboratory reports, radiology reports, and transcribed operative and discharge summaries.

The Spacelabs Inc. physiological monitoring system provides continuous data on cardiovascular and respiratory status on all patients attached to monitors. Ventilators and special-purpose computers (e.g., for respiratory function) are interfaced to the monitors. The Ryder Trauma Center has 40 monitored locations, including resuscitation suites, holding areas, operating rooms, radiology suites, intensive care units, and post-anesthesia recovery units.

The Diatek Inc. Archive anesthesia record management system, which provides computerized anesthesia reporting in each operating room, transfers all its data. These include monitored cardiovascular, respiratory, and anesthetic gas parameters; procedures; notes; drugs administered; and fluid input and output status.

A digital voice management system, developed in-house, allows voice records of operative dictations to be included in the record. Dictation and review of dictations can be done at any telephone. Voice records are handled like any other data source. This permits the production of management reports indicating which patient records must be transcribed or have yet to be dictated. Additionally, other treating clinicians can review a dictated record before it is transcribed.

The last sources of data are images that are digitized, including x-rays, video clips, and photographs. Various personal computer image capture boards are used for this purpose. In the near future, digital x-ray images such as CAT scans will be transferred directly from their source.

The CARE computer system is client/server-based. However, there are two types of client. Most of the nearly 200 workstations in the Ryder Trauma Center are of the first type: alphanumeric color terminals (the Wyse Model 9200). This equipment is relatively inexpensive. Clients of the second type are Microsoft Windows 95 personal computer workstations. The underlying philosophy of the CARE system is to capture and provide clinical information at the point of care. The low cost Wyse "dumb terminals" have allowed the placement of many highly reliable points of interaction with patient data.

The servers are now based on computers from Dell (200 MHz, with single and dual Pentium processors by Intel). The Microsoft NT operating system is used, and there are database servers and application servers. All application and database software was written at the Ryder Trauma Center. Most applications were written in M Technology, of Micronetics. The M Technology database is hierarchical. However, K-B Systems M-SQL was used to map all data to a relational data structure. There are four sets of database servers, each responsible for a logical grouping of data (e.g., laboratory results). Each server has a 10- or 20-gigabyte multiple disk array. Each server pair functions as a primary server and backup server.

If a primary system fails, an operator can make the backup server take on the primary role in a few minutes. If the failed server cannot be brought back on line within an hour, a new computer is loaded with the previous day's archived data and brought into service. The software synchronizes the two databases after a disconnection. Fortunately, this is done while the primary server is on-line supporting clinical functions. Because of this level of redundancy, the CARE system has not been off-line since it become operational with the opening of the Ryder Trauma Center in May 1992. (It is noteworthy that Hurricane Andrew, which hit Miami on August 24, 1992, caused the Ryder Trauma Center to be run on emergency power for 2 weeks. In spite of many power glitches as internal generators came on-line and off-line, the CARE system ran continuously.)

An SQL server by Oracle based on a Compat server, with dual 160 MHz Pentium processors and 20 gigabytes of arrayed disk storage, running the Microsoft NT operating system, provides a high performance research database. This system is automatically updated with data elements of importance to the various research activities from the M-Technology servers. This server also maintains all multimedia data including digitized videos, images, and voice recordings from dictations. This system supports a number of multicenter research programs.

The second type of server is the application server. There are presently six application servers. These servers are also based on Pentium 200 MHz single- and dual-processor computers running the NT operating system and M-Technology software. Each server can support 40 simultaneous terminal clients. All screens and the supporting software reside on these servers. The connection among the various servers is based on an Ethernet physical layer with multiple protocols including NetWare, the Internet protocol TCP/IP, and a proprietary Micronetics data linkage. Terminal servers are distributed throughout the hospital and medical center offices. They connect to the servers through the network and provide virtual connections to each terminal. The terminal servers contain intelligence to determine the load on each application server. They "connect" each terminal to the least occupied application server.

The applications in the CARE system are designed to meet clinical responsibilities, such as writing an admission note or generating a bill for professional services, and to contribute data to a database that can be used for administrative and research purposes. The philosophy is that specific handwritten or dictated documents can be replaced with computer-generated documents. The key is that the treating clinician enters data into a computer workstation at the point of care. At this time, the following functions are performed exclusively on computer workstations:

Procedure note writing
> All non–operating room procedures and some operating room procedures (e.g., negative exploratory laparotomy)
> Nursing admission and daily summaries in resuscitation, recovery, and intensive care

Professional billing
> Operating room
> Intensive care unit

Scheduling and resource management for the operating rooms
Acquisition, storage, and review of multimedia data
> X-rays
> Photographs
> Video
> Voice records (e.g., dictations)

Internet-based teleconferencing for multidisciplinary reviews of clinical or research cases
Delivery of computer-based lectures
Delivery of reference sources such as MEDLINE

The CARE Information System: Applications

The screens displayed in Figures 1.1 to 1.25 outline some of the functionality of the CARE system. Figure 1.1 demonstrates the "sign on" screen. Each user has both a user number and a password. The system allows the limitation of access by applications, patient, and data element. Access can be provided for viewing and/or entering data. When each user identifies himself to the system at the sign on screen, the system will provide access only to the functions approved for that individual.

Figure 1.2 shows the use of menus, which are at the heart of this system. Either moving to a choice with the arrow keys or typing the first letter of a choice's name highlights a choice. Once a choice has been highlighted, the "enter" key brings about the action. Navigational menus such as this display only choices that are permitted for the user. If a user were not permitted to use the trauma registry, the choice REGISTRY would not appear on his menu. In this case the user has highlighted ICU MENU, and pushing the enter key will bring up the ICU menu.

Figure 1.3 shows the ICU menu that an ICU attending physician would see. Each menu item typically takes the user into another menu, with a series of choices or to an end point. There are subsecond response times from one menu to the next. If the menu choice is CENSUS, the end point

```
Copyright, (C), 1996 Jeffrey S. Augenstein, M.D., Ph.D. All Rights Reserved
                     UM/JMMC C.A.R.E. SYSTEM
                          VERSION 2.60




                    ┌─────────────────────────────┐
                    │ USER NUMBER:                │
                    │ PASSWORD:    ▓▓▓▓▓▓▓▓        │
                    └─────────────────────────────┘


    UNDER STATE LAW AND PHT POLICY, UNAUTHORIZED DISCLOSURE OF THE CONFIDENTIAL
    INFORMATION THAT FOLLOWS CAN RESULT IN HOSPITAL AND/OR PROFESSIONAL
    DISCIPLINE, CIVIL LIABILITY AND IN SOME CIRCUMSTANCES CRIMINAL PENALTIES.
    FOR MORE INFORMATION PLEASE REFER TO THE PRIVACY AND CONFIDENTIALITY MANUAL.



               ┌──────────────────────────────────────────┐
               │  C.A.R.E. System Computer Lab ==> 585-1190 │
               └──────────────────────────────────────────┘


                 [ Edit fields - tab to bottom when done ]
```

FIGURE 1.1. Sign-On.

```
AUGENSTEIN    UNIVERSITY OF MIAMI/JACKSON MEMORIAL MEDICAL CENTER    NEWMAIL
                           C.A.R.E. SYSTEM




              ┌────────────────System Menu────────────────┐
              │ ICU  ICU MENU          REG  REGISTRY       │
              │ OFF  OFFICE APPLICATIONS RES  RESUS MENU    │
              │ ORM  OR MENU           TCU  TRAUMA SERVICE  │
              │ REC  RECOVERY MENU                          │
              └────────────────────────────────────────────┘
```

FIGURE 1.2. Main Menu.

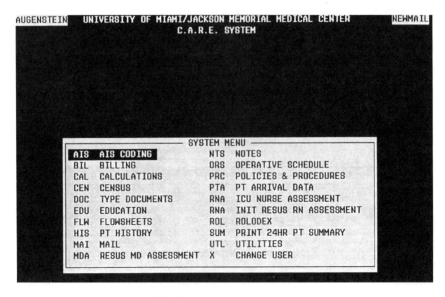

FIGURE 1.3. Trauma Attending Main Menu.

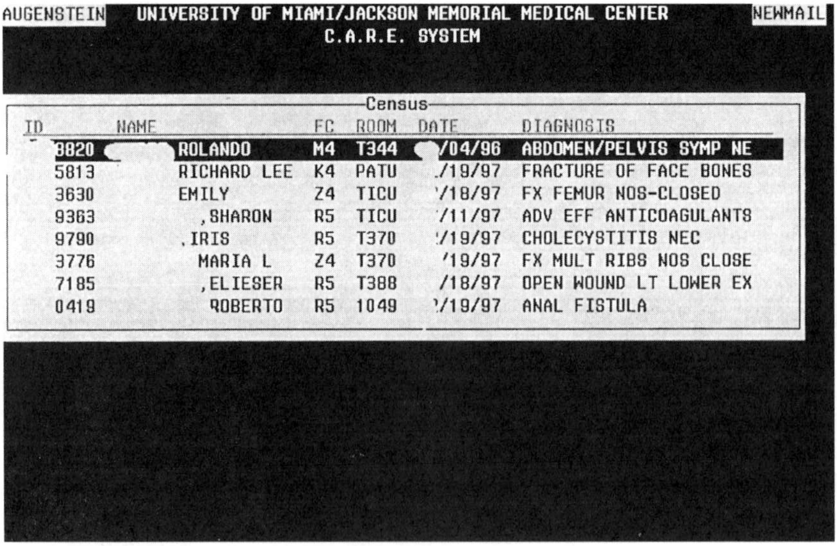

FIGURE 1.4. Census.

shown in Figure 1.4, will appear. If the user desires a different view of the patients, pushing the F1 function key will provide the next screen (Fig. 1.5) which allows the creation of a custom census. This screen provides significant database search capabilities. If desired, however, the user can default to one of the existing censuses by pushing the F1 key on the DEFAULT CENSUS field.

Figure 1.6 shows one page of the options. The various "Crash" choices relate to study censuses. In fact a census can be created for any study. Patients can be in the hospital or discharged. If they are being followed in Jackson clinics, their data (e.g., laboratory studies) will be available on-line in the CARE system.

Once a patient has been chosen, a specific type of clinical data can be entered or reviewed. If FLOWSHEETS was chosen from the ICU attending menu (Fig. 1.3), the next menu would indicate the types of flowsheet available. Figure 1.7 lists the choices. The EVENT FLOWSHEET summarizes all the data in the system in a time-oriented manner. It will combine all data types (e.g., laboratory and radiology reports), placing each on a separate row. If the user chooses LABS FLOWSHEET, the various groups of laboratory tests that have been performed on the patient will be listed (Fig. 1.8). Choosing BLOOD GAS ANALYSIS I will produce the flowsheet shown in Figure 1.9. The flowsheet can be scrolled up and down or right and left with the arrow keys. Any row of data can be viewed in whole-page mode by moving the cursor (via the arrow keys) to the row and pushing the

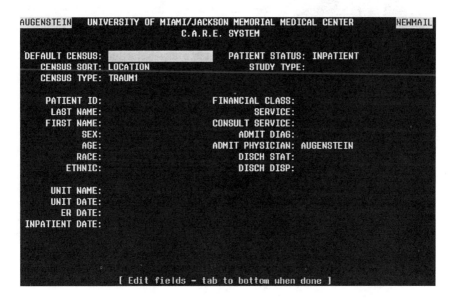

FIGURE 1.5. Custom Census Screen.

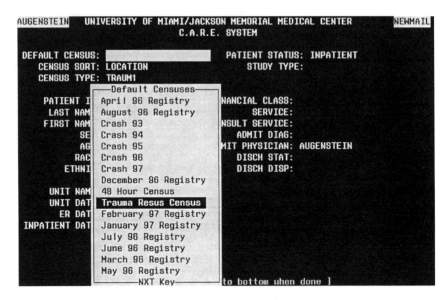

FIGURE 1.6. Default Census Menu.

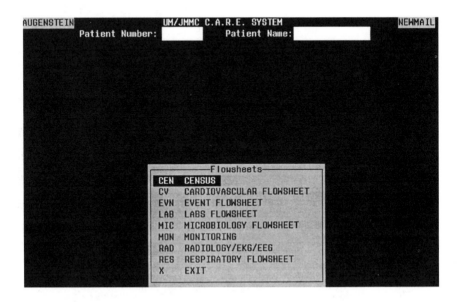

FIGURE 1.7. Flowsheet Menu.

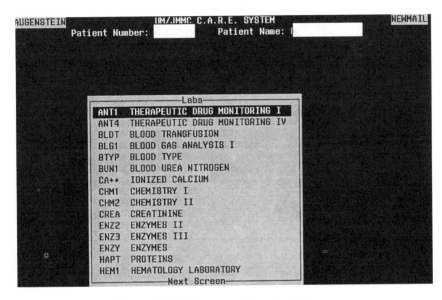

FIGURE 1.8. Laboratory Flowsheet Menu.

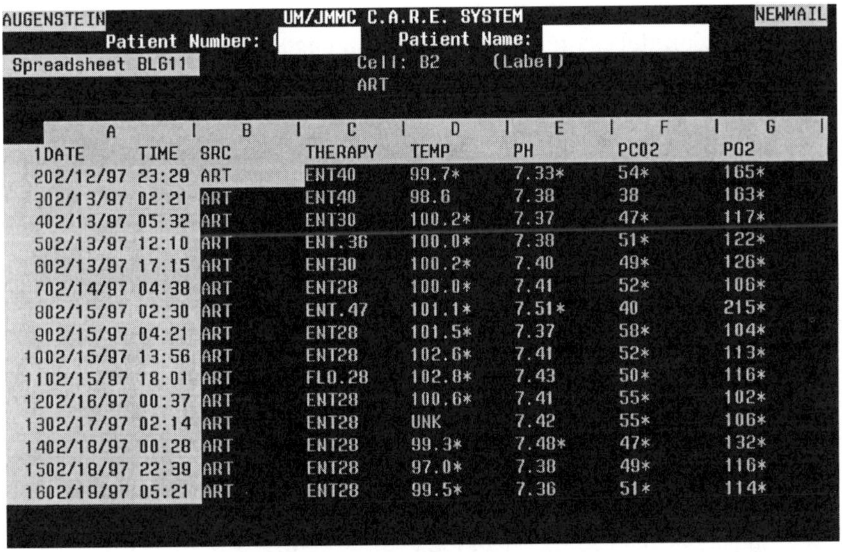

FIGURE 1.9. Blood Gas Flowsheet.

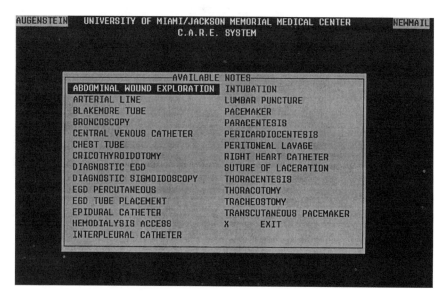

FIGURE 1.10. Procedure Notes Menu.

F3 key. This feature is very useful for test results (e.g., radiology reports). The flowsheet shows only the type of study (e.g., "portable chest x-ray"). The F3 key produces the report. In the full-page mode, the user can scroll through all the reports.

The various note-writing functions in the CARE system are its most used components. Choosing NOTES on the ICU attending menu (Fig. 1.3) brings up the menu shown in Figure 1.10. Choosing CENTRAL VENOUS CATHETER brings up the next form (Fig. 1.11).

The screen presented in Figure 1.11 is typical of the family of procedure notes listed in Figure 1.10, where the user basically fills in the blanks from menu choices. In this case the user has pushed the F1 key while in the "Indication" blank. These notes are created by determining the spectrum of approaches that can be used for a given procedure. Boilerplate text is then provided, with choices left as blanks. There is a continuing evolution of these notes as practices change. However, virtually all procedures not performed in the operating room are documented in this way. A printed copy of the note is placed in the chart. Since printing is such an important part of this record-keeping system, there are laser printers near every terminal.

As illustrated by the completed note given in Figure 1.12, CARE nursing notes list procedures that are performed. These lists provide data to generate daily management reports of missing documentation.

User acceptance of the CARE system has been quite good. In spite of the emphasis on graphic user interfaces in the press, this simple character-based

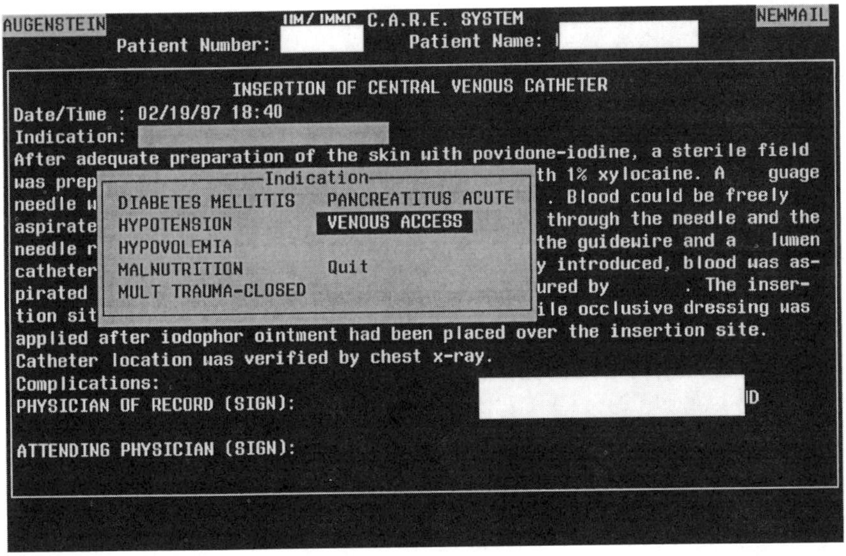

```
AUGENSTEIN         UM/JMMC C.A.R.E. SYSTEM              NEWMAIL
        Patient Number: [      ]    Patient Name: [          ]

              INSERTION OF CENTRAL VENOUS CATHETER
Date/Time : 02/19/97 18:40
Indication: [               ]
After adequate preparation of the skin with povidone-iodine, a sterile field
was prep┌──────────Indication──────────┐th 1% xylocaine. A    guage
needle w│ DIABETES MELLITIS  PANCREATITUS ACUTE │. Blood could be freely
aspirate│ HYPOTENSION      │ VENOUS ACCESS │ through the needle and the
needle r│ HYPOVOLEMIA                    │the guidewire and a   lumen
catheter│ MALNUTRITION       Quit        │y introduced, blood was as-
pirated │ MULT TRAUMA-CLOSED             │ured by      . The inser-
tion sit└──────────────────────────────┘ile occlusive dressing was
applied after iodophor ointment had been placed over the insertion site.
Catheter location was verified by chest x-ray.
Complications:
PHYSICIAN OF RECORD (SIGN):              [              ]D

ATTENDING PHYSICIAN (SIGN):
```

FIGURE 1.11. Central Venous Catheter Note-Indications Menu.

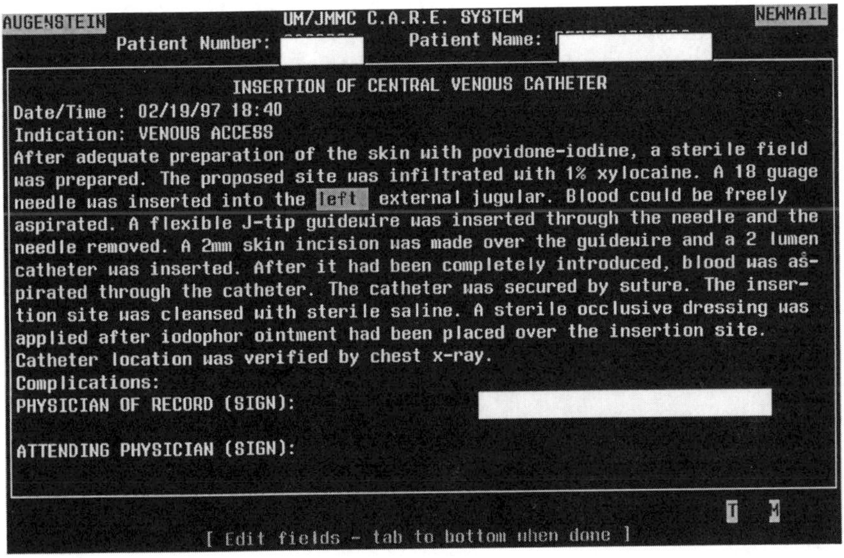

```
AUGENSTEIN         UM/JMMC C.A.R.E. SYSTEM              NEWMAIL
        Patient Number: [      ]    Patient Name: [          ]

              INSERTION OF CENTRAL VENOUS CATHETER
Date/Time : 02/19/97 18:40
Indication: VENOUS ACCESS
After adequate preparation of the skin with povidone-iodine, a sterile field
was prepared. The proposed site was infiltrated with 1% xylocaine. A 18 guage
needle was inserted into the left external jugular. Blood could be freely
aspirated. A flexible J-tip guidewire was inserted through the needle and the
needle removed. A 2mm skin incision was made over the guidewire and a 2 lumen
catheter was inserted. After it had been completely introduced, blood was as-
pirated through the catheter. The catheter was secured by suture. The inser-
tion site was cleansed with sterile saline. A sterile occlusive dressing was
applied after iodophor ointment had been placed over the insertion site.
Catheter location was verified by chest x-ray.
Complications:
PHYSICIAN OF RECORD (SIGN):              [              ]

ATTENDING PHYSICIAN (SIGN):

              [ Edit fields - tab to bottom when done ]
```

FIGURE 1.12. Completed Central Venous Catheter Note.

menuing interface has not been a limitation. Perhaps simplicity is its strength. At this time most of our users are not particularly interested in computers. They just want to do a job. If the system eases a task, it will be used. This has been particularly true for intensive care unit nursing initial and shift-based assessments. The time for documentation has decreased from about an hour to 10 minutes. The quality of the documentation improved in the process.

The strategy over the next 2 years is to continue to deploy the terminal workstations in most clinical environments. Because of interest in the hospital at large, the CARE system has been expanded into all the operating rooms, labor and delivery, the cardiac catherization laboratories, the Department of Neurological Surgery, and the total transplantation program. The CARE system is scheduled to expand to 600 terminal workstations by the end of 1997. Certain applications, however, warrant a graphic user interface. A group of projects are in place that put a Microsoft Windows 95 interface on certain parts of the CARE system.

The main Windows effort is CrashCARE, which is used to specifically study patients injured in automobile crashes, is a typical client/server application. The client software, in Microsoft's VisualBasic, is fairly extensive and must run on high level personal computers. The data are maintained on the previously described SQL server.

CrashCARE adds some unique functionality to the CARE system, including a very detailed injury description methodology, multimedia data management, and a graphic database-querying capability. Figure 1.13 demonstrates the first part of the injury description module. When the user points with the mouse to a part of the body, in this case the anterior left abdomen, a list of types of injury to this area appears on the screen.

Figure 1.14 demonstrates that the "Contusion/Bruise, Left Abdomen" has been added to the list of injuries. By double clicking on that injury marker, the user can obtain additional detail. Figure 1.15 shows the choices that are presented. The user then identifies the general system that was injured, responding via the pop-up menu. If the user chooses ORGANS, a prompt with organs that reside in that region will appear, as shown in Figure 1.16. If SPLEEN is selected, the parts of that organ will be listed, as shown in Figure 1.17. These terms come from SNOMED III, a very detailed nomenclature system developed over a 30-year period by the American College of Pathologists.

Next the user has the opportunity to identify the type of injury to the spleen. Questions are typically grouped so that the injury can be classified into an appropriate AIS severity level. The concept is that when clinicians begin to describe injuries in the resuscitation phase of care, the injury description can be refined as further definition becomes available. The injury list is available to any clinician writing a note about the patient. It is hoped that this feature will reduce the number of erroneous descriptions of injuries that often appear in charts. To date the injuries of over a thousand severely injured patients have been described with this system.

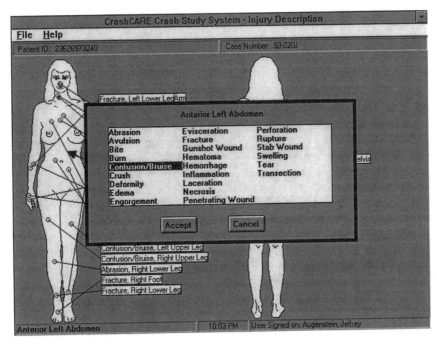

FIGURE 1.13. Injury Description Screen—Injury Type Menu.

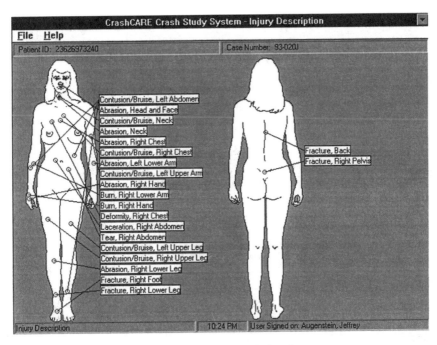

FIGURE 1.14. Injury Description Screen.

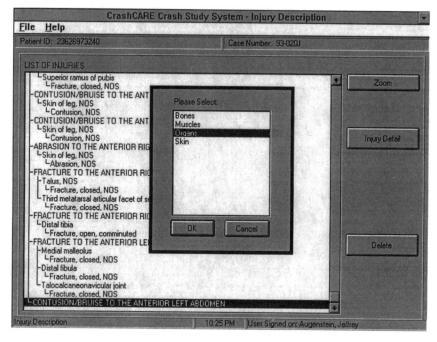

FIGURE 1.15. Injury Description Test Screen—Location Menu.

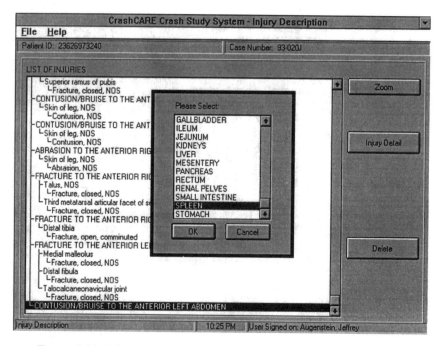

FIGURE 1.16. Injury Description Text Screen—General Anatomy Menu.

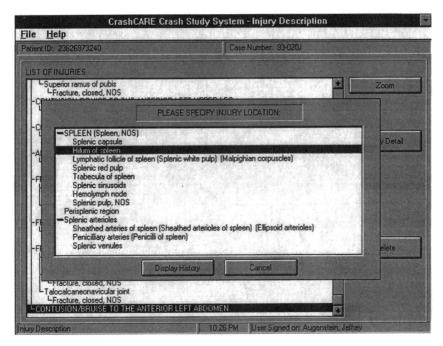

FIGURE 1.17. Injury Description Text Screen—Specific Anatomy Menu.

The system translates each injury to an ICD-9 and AIS 90 code for professional billing and quality assurance purposes, utilizing software developed as the Tricode product. Figure 1.18 shows the translation screen. The "Search ICD-9" and "Search AIS" functions present electronic versions of each coding manual for experts to override the computer's decisions. This screen also provides a connection between injuries and the automobile contacts that are hypothesized to have caused them.

CrashCARE provides applications to acquire, describe, store, and retrieve multimedia data objects including digitized data from x-rays, photographs, voice recordings, and video segments, as well as three-dimensional animations. Figure 1.19 shows a multipanel display. The user, who picked these objects out of a larger list, was able to configure the juxtaposition of the various objects and easily make rearrangements. A single large view of any item can be presented by double clicking an individual panel.

CrashCARE provides a simple way for those who are not database experts to analyze virtually all the data elements in the CrashCARE system. The challenge is that this type of database is constructed from many separate tables. The connection between tables, such as one that holds injuries and one that contains hospital costs, may be complex. Instead of one-to-one connections, there are often many-to-one or many-to-many. The database analysis system contains all the knowledge about the tables and their connections. The system fills in that expertise after the user has posed an

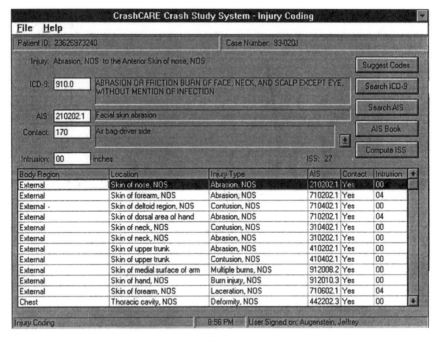

FIGURE 1.18. Injury Coding Screen.

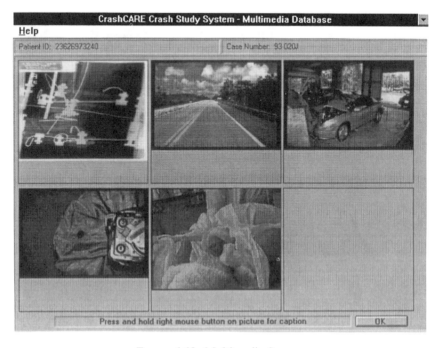

FIGURE 1.19. Multimedia Screen.

analysis. Figure 1.20 demonstrates the first screen in a typical database query. This screen determines the starting point for the query. In this case the user has chosen "injury" and additionally has pointed to "Abdomen" with the mouse.

Next the system will determine which injuries to the abdomen are to be analyzed. "Liver" was chosen from a list (the same used in describing the injuries) of the components of the abdomen. The system returns all the parts of the liver uniquely described in the database in Figure 1.21.

The user can then name additional criteria for the search. Figure 1.22 shows the addition of the criterion "Airbag" = "Frontal Deployed" to the liver injury criterion, and Figure 1.23 shows the two criteria being ANDed together. The report-generating choices (Fig. 1.24) request the names of columns to appear in the spreadsheet it will create. The highlighted items will be displayed as columns on the spreadsheet.

The spreadsheet as designed appears in Figure 1.25. The results of a database query could be placed in other applications (e.g., statistical analysis programs, other databases). However, the spreadsheet seems to be the most popular recipient.

The CARE Information System: Future Directions

At this time the Ryder Trauma Center with the CARE system provides a laboratory for the study of the impact of computerized information management on a complex acute care environment. Future directions are based on perceived needs, technological possibilities, and funding support. The following lessons have been learned to date in this trauma information management project.

An internal team of software and hardware experts can develop and maintain a mission-critical information system. (Currently 10 full-time personnel, of whom seven are programmers, support the CARE and CrashCARE systems; over 300 terminals and printers are connected directly to the system.)

Clinicians of all types, including department chairmen and operating room nurses, can and will use the system proficiently.

Physicians and nurses will use management information in decision making. They will continuously demand more information. To get needed data, they will encourage the computerization of functions (e.g., note writing), and operating room scheduling is a by-product of the production of needed management information.

The CARE system generates hundreds of management reports each month. Some are produced daily. Nearly 20% of the CARE team's work effort is devoted to generating management and research reports. Virtually all the trauma center's quality assurance and registry reports are generated by computer.

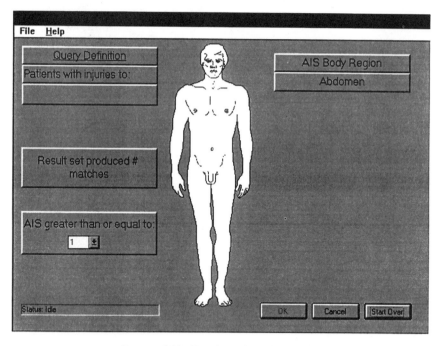

FIGURE 1.20. Database Search Screen.

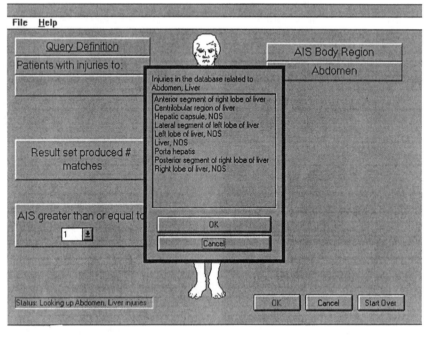

FIGURE 1.21. Database Search Screen—Unique Injuries List.

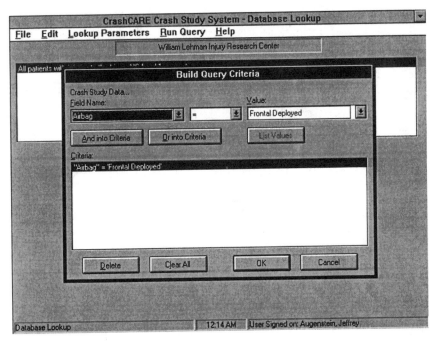

FIGURE 1.22. Build Query Screen—Criteria.

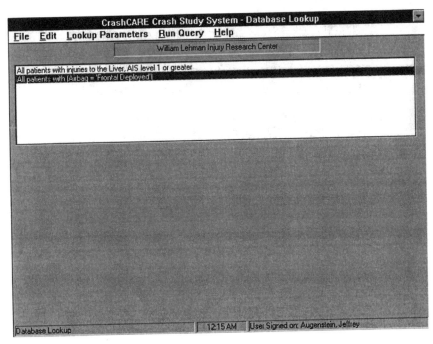

FIGURE 1.23. Build Query Screen—Criteria Combination.

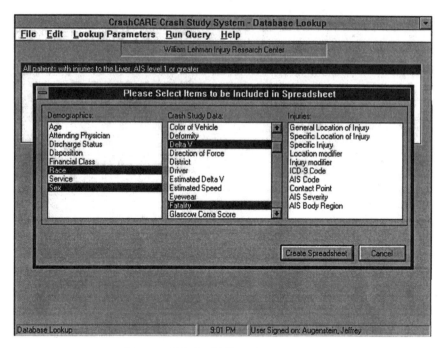

FIGURE 1.24. Build Flowsheet Screen.

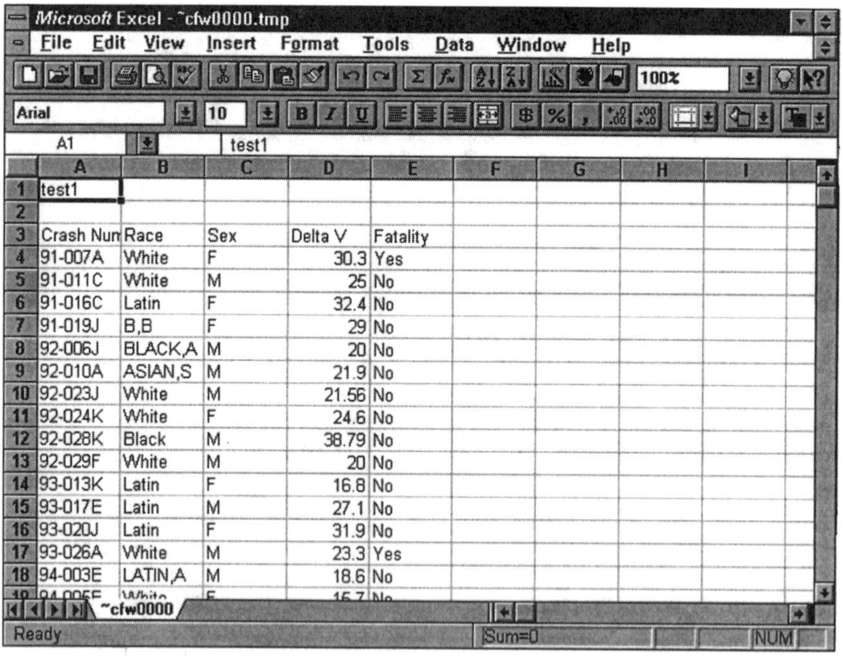

FIGURE 1.25. Flowsheet.

The next phase involves continued deployment of new applications and the study of the impact of the systems on performance at the trauma center. A combined intensive care flowsheet with orders and Kardex module, based on bedside workstations, is in final testing with the Windows 95 user interface on personal computers. Following that implementation, the orders system will be deployed throughout the center via the CARE terminals.

Research projects are in place to determine if wireless (radiolinked) terminals and speech recognition can be used to augment the functionality of the CARE system. Movable workstations seem to be needed to fully support note-writing and orders' management on the two ward floors. Clearly, voice recognition would facilitate the entry of text-intensive components of notes such as observations in an operating room. (These two technologies have been under evaluation for the last 6 years and appear to be becoming adequately functional and affordable.)

The main regret at this time is our past inability to devote resources to the evaluation of the impact of information management technology on the performance of the trauma center. With cooperation of the University of Miami graduate programs in nursing and engineering, three graduate student research initiatives are in place and are expected to provide analyzable results by the end of 1997.

The first program employs operations research techniques, to identify situations that could be dangerous in the event that critical information was unavailable or miscommunicated. The study is modeling the flow of important information about the patient (e.g., allergy history, medication administration) as the patient is transferred from resuscitation to the operating room and the intensive care unit. The goal is to develop applications that assure the correct and timely transfer of information.

The second graduate student study is aimed at analyzing the accuracy of description in the traditional paper chart as a baseline for the implementation of computer applications. The initial study is evaluating the description of injuries. In this study, patients' injuries are independently observed and described by clinical experts. The patients' charts are critically evaluated to determine the completeness, timeliness, accuracy, and consistency of references to injuries during each patient's hospitalization.

The third graduate study involves the development of a usability laboratory to evaluate the acceptability and functionality of new applications. This work is concentrating on the evaluation of the newly developed intensive care bedside flowsheet, orders, and Kardex modules. Nurses and physicians will be presented with patient scenarios requiring the entry or analysis of data in this system. Accuracy, time and motion of the activities, and attitudes about using this module (instead of the present paper approach) will all be evaluated.

In summary, the CARE system development project at the Ryder Trauma Center has provided an important opportunity to address the improvement in trauma care delivery through better information management. Clearly much more needs to be done in analyzing the care environment, developing systems to meet perceived needs, and studying the ongoing process of care delivery in a rapidly changing clinical world.

Section II

2
Informatics in Prehospital Care

M. JACK LEE, ANTHONY J. MARTINEZ, LETICIA M. RUTLEDGE, AND KIMBALL I. MAULL

The importance of informatics in the prehospital setting is just emerging as the driving forces change within the emergency medical services (EMS) industry. Modern EMS has its roots in battlefield emergency care and related experiences of the Korean and Vietnam wars. During the early 1960s and 1970s, the EMS mission was to strive to provide advanced emergency trauma and cardiac care to the public regardless of cost. The media and television sitcoms heightened the public's awareness of "paramedicine." Ideas based largely on anecdotal and deductive reasoning led to the prehospital application of emergency care techniques previously confined to the hospital emergency room. EMS services proliferated and ran the spectrum from small rural volunteer fire departments to large for-profit, big city private EMS providers. However, because the focus was on filling a void in the cascade of patient care, the need for data and information collection was not fully recognized until two to three decades later. Our society has evolved to a high level of medical sophistication and performance expectations and, as a result, informatics is essential for surviving in today's changing EMS world.

Informatics in Early EMS

Just, over two decades ago, if someone asked the owner of an ambulance service what type of information was required to get the job done, the answer would probably have been none or very little. The early EMS providers gathered information almost exclusively for the purposes of patient billing. Regions that were fortunate enough to have some type of governing EMS agency or board generally required additional information, most of which was ably handled by the company secretary, and certainly was tabulated without the aid of a computer. Beyond billing information, most services kept records to verify that vehicles met local standards, if these existed. Records on current provider certification, usually at the EMT-Basic level, were also kept to meet local requirements. In the early

1970s, concepts like continuing education (CE) and quality assurance (QA) were still a few years off. The mom-and-pop services of the 1960s and early 1970s, in most regions, were more concerned with their day-to-day existence as medical taxi services.

However, the 1970s were also a time for change in EMS. Public services and some of the larger private providers began to promulgate the concept of advanced EMTs and/or paramedics. Mobile intensive care units (MICUs), combined with enhanced expectations based on trauma care practiced in Korea and Vietnam, culminated in the gradual establishment of advanced EMS systems throughout the United States. Data on highway traffic fatalities and other reports supported the need to respond more effectively to trauma and the threat of sudden death from cardiac arrest. Paramedics arrived on the scene in full force by the late 1970s and with them brought new demands for informatics in the prehospital setting.

Informatics and Paramedicine

Through the training and use of paramedical personnel, protocols had to be developed by physicians to regulate what, how, and when advanced cardiac and trauma care would be delivered in the field. Early paramedic systems had strict protocols compared to the services today. Data were required to monitor this new and widely expanding field of medicine. Data concerning training and procedure utilization for license renewal and/or recertification had to be kept by services to meet local medical control standards as well as requirements of bodies such as state regulatory agencies. Services providing advanced life support (ALS) care began to need full-time training officers to provide the education and quality assurance necessary to keep pace with the rapidly changing environment of EMS. The changing scope of practice and the need for data collection are but two examples of requirements to justify providing advanced life support in a given area. New procedures and protocols depended on educational in-services and monitoring of the new treatment regimens over time. In addition, services assumed a responsibility to ensure and verify competency of the employees working for them.

The Driving Force: Medical Direction

A key player in the success of any prehospital system is the committed medical director. As EMS evolved, the medical director's role became increasingly complex and increased the need for information accordingly. All aspects of EMS are directly related to medical direction informatics. Examples include medical priority dispatch systems (MPDS), system protocols, and the quality assurance process. The concept of active medical direction is dependent on active involvement in the quality assurance process. Field and classroom observation provide some indication of personnel's overall performance. Yet motivating capable prehospital care providers demands timely evaluation of actual hands-on patient care, together with appropriate feedback. Reliable data are critical. Such information can then be used for educational reinforcement based on actual patient care for the purpose of improving patient care. Informatics-based education and quality assurance programs establish a logical linkage between classroom instruction and field care. As a result, the focal point of prehospital informatics is how it is utilized in quality assurance and the verification of competency.

Informatics and Quality Assurance

High performance EMS systems are in need of mechanisms to constantly monitor the effectiveness of patient care delivery. To remain competitive in today's prehospital marketplace, these systems must maintain the highest levels of performance.

The key to the effective use of informatics in the quality assurance setting is usable and meaningful data. The information must be accessible and usable in standard formats. Cross-compatibility makes baseline data available for several different projects. The data elements can be used concurrently by several different groups.

Injury type and severity are simple examples of data elements. The initial data provide baseline elements that can be used from system response through rehabilitation, and ultimately to a patient's return to a functional role in society. Following a patient from injury to discharge is becoming a reality as a result of the cooperative efforts among providers within the trauma care system.

Another area is coding the prehospital care provider's provisional diagnosis for recovery/billing purposes, that is, applying the International Classification of Disease codes, ninth revision (ICD-9) for this function. The dynamic changes brought on by managed care are placing even greater demands on hospitals in the area of validating patient care and transport based on medical necessity. Accurate and timely completion and submission of reports with data elements that can be used by all members of the patient care system are vital components for success in our rapidly changing health care system.

Both operational and clinical data elements are necessary to indicate the level of performance of an agency. Operational data elements include vehicle performance, including available service hours and downtime hours. Additionally, all aspects of response time criteria are now available as a result of the advances in computer technology. Complete categorization of the types of call received facilitates a comparison between the initial call type and the actual call type based on arrival data and patient evaluation.

Treatment modalities are also compiled in an effort to monitor trends over time. For example, advanced airway procedures can be monitored from several perspectives. Individual, agency, and system performance can all be monitored in this fashion. More importantly, individual report elements are also linked to advanced airway management, so individual reports can be pulled for case review.

Hospital transports and diverting of transporting units are related directly to the efficiency of an EMS system. Response times are directly related to timely availability of EMS units, and a large percentage of diverts could impact timely response time.

Cardiac arrest management data elements include all phases of total call time. Additionally, protocol compliance and procedure success elements are readily available for trending by provider, by service, and within the system.

Emergent transport to hospital facilitates a comparison of prehospital impressions of injury severity with hospital severity of injury scores.

Furthermore, trauma triage protocol elements are also readily available for trending. As with cardiac arrest calls, all elements of total call time are readily available. In particular, uncomplicated scene times on trauma calls are expected to be under 10 minutes. In an effort to facilitate the administration of timely and efficient prehospital care, EMS product manufacturers have continually provided the EMS system with equipment and adjuncts that require testing and must have data to support their usage.

Informatics and Prehospital Research/Training

Prehospital research began with paramedicine. Initially, the research was used to test and find new ways to provide prehospital cardiac life support, such as the studies performed in Seattle concerning CPR and sudden death. Response time criteria related to EMS system structure are still heavily influenced by these data.

However, other procedures and modes of equipment use remained based on tradition and anecdotal reports—not all of them unbiased. Advanced airway management was first studied with data gathered by manufacturers of products like the Gordon-Don Michael Esophageal Obturator Airway (EOA), Early studies reported equivalence in the respective ability to oxygenate a patient of the EOA and endotracheal intubation.[13,14] Later, nonbiased studies revealed the device to be less efficacious than the time-honored practice of intubation.[15,20] Data and the application of information technologies in EMS were necessary to arrive at these conclusions.

In addition to early research, information technology took on a new role in EMS—training adjuncts.

Training aids such as computerized cardiac rhythm generators became commonplace in the early 1980s, to the point that most large services could afford to have one available for advanced cardiac life support (ACLS) classes. These tools became available to paramedics in addition to their core curriculum. As simulators became more sophisticated, they became programmable to better simulate a complete cardiac care scenario. With the proliferation of personal computers, full cardiac scenario simulations were developed to provide a means of education apart from the traditional classroom. Increased education and quality assurance activities eventually led to the use of the PC to gather and analyze the increasing amounts of data concerning procedures, confirmation of protocols, and the like. EMS medical directors were beginning to ask for hard evidence of skill maintenance and continuing education requirements.

In addition, local authorities began to request information to verify a service's compliance with established standards. An example of such a standard was response time verification. An example of the use of information technologies in EMS dispatch began effectively in the mid-1980s with the ETAK Mobile Navigator system and Computer-Aided Dispatch (CAD) system, both of which allow services to gather real-time data concerning call dispatch times and mileage with the aid of a computerized automatic vehicle location (AVL) tracking system. The ETAK AVL system allowed dispatchers to see the location of units throughout the city on a map screen. Upon receiving a call in the dispatch center, the dispatcher could type the call into the CAD and an icon showing the call location would appear on the screen. It became a simple matter to select the closest unit to the call with the visual aid of the CAD and thereby begin to effectively reduce response times.

Prior to the CAD, most response time data had to be entered into a PC from handwritten dispatch radio log files. The use of informatics by dispatch centers provided a tremendous advance in data availability to EMS providers. Dispatch data and educational data gave the EMS quality assurance manager new tools to better provide reports to medical control concerning the status of their organizations.

Use of Data to Meet New Industry Challenges

Today EMS providers are affected by competition, turf wars, and the shrinking availability of funds. The EMS provider in the 1990s is challenged by increasing costs and decreasing reimbursement, with the result that services are obliged to operate more efficiently. Likewise, traditional EMS practices are being challenged as insurance and third-party payers begin to question the need for such services. EMS agencies must do original research and gather data to validate their practices and support their need to exist in the face of health care reform. Informatics has taken on a new and expanded role in EMS today. Early on in EMS, information technologies were largely limited to education. Training aids, mannequins, and computerized simulators for ACLS, the cornerstone for EMS, were the main uses of such technology. The 1980s proved the need for information technology in EMS call management. CAD and AVL were being used to aid in the application of new EMS management concepts like system status management (SSM), first reported by Stout.[21] System status management was the first true use of informatics in EMS. Using queuing theory as a basis for deployment, call data were gathered to plot zones of high priority call probabilities for each hour of the day, every day of the week. The resulting SSM plan allowed services to operate more efficiently by proving the value of peak-load staffing based on detailed data analyses. Applied properly, SSM can effectively reduce response times by strategically placing units at mobile posts based on the deployment schema from the informatics data.

Throughout the industry, services began to report significant reductions in response time, making them more competitive in the growing environment of mergers and takeovers. Ideas like SSM brought about new positions in EMS such as the system status manager, a person devoted to data collection and refinement of the services SSM plan. The institution of such planning was not without its problems. Strict application of the early ideas of SSM usually meant that units worked harder as services used peak-load staffing to streamline their costs.

A more gentle approach came from applying further data analysis called unit hour utilization (UHU), which takes into account the average workload for each vehicle on the street. A UHU of 0.40 meant that on average the unit spent 40 minutes out of every 100 minutes on a call. Targeting ideal UHUs when designing staffing patterns allows for a more cost-effective way to apply the concepts of SSM to EMS.

Although SSM is used largely by private providers, some public utility models are starting to examine it as a means of responding to cuts in their funding. Fire fighting unions, facing the reality of improved fire codes and decreasing need for fire suppression man power, turn to EMS as a means of job security and continued funding from public coffers. Careful application of SSM alone could not protect private services from being challenged by public providers who see EMS as the way to continued existence. Private providers have turned to prehospital research to answer questions ranging from the need for specific EMS response configurations to the use of automatic defibrillators on fire trucks followed by ALS transport (usually by a private provider).

Clearly, more data are needed to answer the questions on type and level of services to provide in the prehospital setting. In the 1980s and early 1990s, registries of data that involved EMS began to emerge. Registries of specialized data were formed to validate and verify the application of continually developing concepts such as trauma centers and the role of EMS in a large trauma system. Hospital trauma registries often utilized specialized data to match prehospital and hospital data, providing a more complete clinical picture of patients and their total care in the system.

Hospital Trauma and Prehospital Data

Because hospital trauma registries are not usually population based, trauma data collected in hospitals cover only the more seriously injured patients requiring hospital admission. Although limited, trauma registries are used as a patient care quality improvement tool for hospitals, and this concept can be readily extended to the prehospital environment. Clinically based injury assessment scores can serve as quality assurance indicators to determine preventable or nonpreventable morbidity and mortality. While hospital trauma registries can give a good picture of local trends and clinical issues pertinent to a particular hospital and the prehospital services that transport patients to that hospital, a systems trauma registry provides a larger perspective of trauma incidence, care, and outcome. Likewise, a prehospital service can do a good audit of its own local runs but may not have a systems perspective of what EMS is doing in other parts of the state.

The systems registry, usually a compilation of data from designated trauma centers or, in some states, from all hospitals admitting emergency patients, can link with other systems or state data sources. Examples include databases reported from the statewide EMS run report and traffic crash reporting systems, as well as hospital information discharge data, and the records of the Office of the Medical Investigator, to provide a fuller picture of trauma.

In the near future, all prehospital providers will be able to enter their patient care information into a vehicle-stationed computer, for electronic transmission and downloading into a receiving hospital's emergency department. The data will be uploaded into the hospital's inpatient mainframe system or, if the patient dies, will pass straight to the Office of the Medical Investigator. Duplication will be reduced and, more importantly, pertinent information will be transferred. The continuum of patient care will be both documented and evaluable. The quality assurance loop will be appropriately closed.

Linking trauma registries with prehospital and other data sources provides multiple opportunities for health providers, patients, and the community. Data linkage offers the opportunity for improving standard patient care, provides data for clinical and epidemiological research, and makes accessible to the public information that can be used for local, statewide, and national injury prevention projects.

The use of computerized charting systems will aid both hospital and prehospital information systems by providing computerized data gathering from the providers directly, thereby minimizing error in translation from the documents formerly handwritten by quality assurance personnel.

Use of Informatics in Patient Care: A Case Study in the Use of Informatics to Improve Productivity in a Large Private Metropolitan EMS System

Use of Informatics in Dispatch and Patient Billing

The Albuquerque Ambulance Service (AAS), a large metropolitan, hospital-owned ambulance service in Albuquerque, New Mexico, began using computerized information technology in 1984. Handwritten dispatch logs were entered into an 8-bit personal computer (Tandy SX 100) in Lotus 123 spreadsheet format, to perform descriptive statistical analyses on call types and response times by hour of the day. These early reports allowed AAS to refine unit deployments and provided a means of verifying service performance through careful data gathering and analysis.

This humble beginning in the information age soon expanded to virtually every aspect of the organization. The next 12 years yielded tremendous benefit from properly applying informatics to generate EMS business solutions. In 1986 AAS management personnel appreciated the potential of in-vehicle navigation combined with computer-aided dispatching and automatic vehicle locating and implemented a pilot program of all these new concepts at AAS. Believing that dollars spent wisely on high technology in the areas of data gathering and data reporting can be offset readily through improved efficiency, the program's originators made AAS one of the first EMS systems in the country to utilize full-scale in-vehicle navigation with CAD. Indeed, the application of computerized information systems to the call routing and dispatch functions actually saved the company enough money to cover the cost of the system in its first year of operation. CAD and AVL meant that AAS could perform detailed data analyses far beyond the earlier crude attempts to meet response times with more personnel but without such a system.

The CAD system was upgraded in 1993 with new software that allowed for improved data gathering. This upgrade, along with improvements in peak-load staffing, aided in streamlining the SSM plan. Since 1986, the use of a fully computerized dispatch center and in-vehicle navigation put AAS in the forefront of data analysis, process verification, and refinement in EMS. Still the vision continued in 1990, with the computerization and restructuring of an antiquated billing system.

In 1990 the billing operation underwent further refinement. A server utilizing a metropolis database and state-of-the-art electronic billing and patient account management software (MEDOCUR) was put into place. The hardware consisted of an RS232 serial local area network (LAN) with

Wyse terminals at each of the account manager's desks. Just as the decision to move to computerized dispatch turned out to be profitable, the LAN too caused AAS to realize a gain through a near doubling of cash flow compared to the hand-file paper billing system used previously. High technology now implemented in both dispatch and billing allowed AAS to expand its operation and pay off all back debt to the parent corporation without an increase in cost to the consumer. It was the possible implementation of the new billing system that made the CAD upgrade, and in this advantageous environment, organizational strategic planning turned to other ways to improve operational productivity with information technology.

Use of Informatics in Patient Care Documentation Systems

Over the past few years, both hardware and software have been developed for getting information and documenting patient care delivered in the prehospital setting. Most of the patient care documentation systems (PCDS) are pen-based and utilize an electronic penlike stylus to enter the data onto a laptop or notebook computer. Some use a computerized tablet or similar device that a paramedic can take along to the scene of a call. Pen-based systems often use Microsoft for Pen Computing, or they may have a proprietary MSDOS or similar operating-system-based application for the user interface. For some PCDS the user writes with a pen on a virtual notepad and the system either converts the handwritten report into editable text via optical charter recognition (OCR) or simply stores the handwritten document as a bitmap. Other PCDS use the pen stylus as a pointing device to pick data out of a list of multiple charting alternatives.

Although many products are available, they have not realized their full market potential. Thus EMS system directors may be skeptical of the capacity of the present technology to replace the written patient care record. Paramedics often complain that computerized systems do not write out reports as detailed as they can produce manually. Complex PCDS, with large data sets, may actually require more time to complete than their handwritten predecessors.

Most PCDS are "ruggedized" for field use. However, concerns about theft and damage through abuse and heavy usage are likely to make some EMS directors avoid taking the plunge into computerized charting.

The standards on what constitutes "ruggedized" hardware vary from manufacturer to manufacturer. Services planning to upgrade to fully computerized PCDS, therefore, need to comparison-shop the hardware, doing both speed and durability testing before making a large-scale purchase. Maintenance agreements are a must for high volume, heavily used services.

Total upgrade cost is still another factor in deciding to move to computerized charting. Most PCDS hardware–software combination packages cost between $3000 and $6000 each, depending on the exact hardware and software configurations selected.

Some companies offer only the software. While this may initially seem to be an attractive solution, a purchaser who has attempted to match the right hardware to bargain-priced software to control costs may be left with an inadequate system. When possible, select hardware that has a proven track record, to avoid the expense of having to replace the system sooner than planned. Any move to computerized charting should be preceded by an overall cumulative cost comparison between companies offering combination packages and vendors that sell hardware and software separately. Software that is designed for multiple hardware systems is more desirable than highly proprietary packages.

In addition, companies are responding to the references for "open architecture" in the construction of the latest versions of software. Some companies now offer software with an optional hardware package. The optional hardware solution is attractive to managers of EMS systems with existing hardware who desire to improve or upgrade their software packages. Improving standards will make this latter alternative more viable for most companies and should eventually lead to lower product costs through increased volume in the EMS marketplace.

Unfortunately, the high cost of hardware and software usually limits PCDS to large urban or metropolitan EMS operations. Even so, few large organizations have begun computerized charting even when they can afford a total changeover. The problem with moving to computerized PCDS has been the lack of true industry standards. A standard EMS data set has only recently begun to be defined, in one form or another. Through the efforts of the National Highway Traffic Safety Administration's workshops and committees on standardizing EMS data, a minimum data set has been proposed for systems wishing to participate in data sharing and linkage with other agencies. The move to develop such a standard is driven largely by the desire to facilitate the linkage of EMS data sets with other medical and nonmedical data for clinical and demographic research into traffic crashes and similar traumatic injuries throughout the United States. Many states are participating in a research project with NHTSA called CODES (crash outcome data evaluation system), concerning automobile crash outcomes and their effects both clinically and financially in a given region. Other states have started to adopt this NHTSA minimum data set as the basis for data linkage on projects similar to or modeled after the NHTSA CODES initiative. Software vendors moving to adopt the minimum data set should have a distinct advantage over competitors utilizing a proprietary independent data set.

Minimum EMS data sets offer the ability for EMS agencies to do benchmarking in both clinical and financial areas as well. Data linkage with hospitals and rehabilitation centers allows for the study of outcomes across the trauma care continuum. Prevention programs could have access to clinical data to test, verify, or simply propose a course of action to ameliorate an observable problem. Hard data can be given to legislatures when new laws to protect individuals from injury are proposed. Standardization of data sets can allow different computer hardware and software vendors to compete openly in the EMS market, while maintaining standards for data collection that allow for cross-platform communication, data sharing, and warehousing. Increased competition could lead to reduced cost through the operation of the laws of supply and demand. Increased use of computerized PCDS would have a tremendous impact on all aspects of prehospital medicine.

Quality assurance officers in EMS could have data entered by paramedics at the point of occurrence, allowing for easier data grouping, statistical analyses, and interpretation. With the old systems, quality improvement (QI) officers and their staffs often labor for hours, reading handwritten charts and typing the data into spreadsheets or databases for analysis. Deciphering different individuals' handwriting, often from poor quality carbon copies or photocopies of original reports has led to lost or misinterpreted data.

Handwritten reports have little direct structure, and their quality may be influenced by fatigue or, sometimes, an out-and-out aversion to the task. Some paramedics have expressed the belief that only verbal turnover reports and minimal written documentation should be required. Some systems have opted for simple check box sheets to minimize the amount of time and data needed to complete a report. However, as most QI officers will agree, data are necessary to adequately evaluate both individual and system performance. Standardized data sets are needed to adequately compare performance to established standards for EMS. Unfortunately, QI officers often spend considerable time counseling employees on how to chart legibly and completely, leaving less time for actual data analysis. Because of lost, missing, or misread data, evaluations of clinical thresholds are of marginal reliability at best.

Computerized charting, on the other hand, is structured, modal as necessary, and legible. The data are entered into the system by the individuals directly involved in the patient care. QI officers and administrators need only to be able to aggregate the data, do an analysis, and generate reports. More time can be spent on data interpretation as opposed to data entry. The ability to test assumptions current to today's practice more readily and efficiently is both timely and necessary in the face of rising health care costs and shrinking EMS dollars.

The management team at AAS realized early on that data used to properly manage a modified system status (SSM) plan allows the service to maximize cost efficiency by putting the right amount of unit hours on the street. The data from the dispatch CAD and vehicle navigators allows for detailed refinement of the system status plan, deploying units to the high probability call areas and therefore reducing response time.

Use of Informatics for Navigation and Database Building

EMS administrators who have the foresight and ability to use informatics to improve operations and reduce operating costs at the same time will provide leadership for the future. AAS is continuing in its effective use of high technology and informatics systems through the addition of computerized patient charting linked to a newly developed in-vehicle navigation system to replace the current efficient yet aging system.

Data Burst Technologies, with home offices in Kansas City, Missouri, and ETAK in Palo Alto, California, have combined their efforts to build Data Burst's new TouchNav navigation system for AAS. EMS Southwest, a New Mexico corporation, is providing the PCDS software EMS ChartWriter 2000 and an accompanying QI software data management solution. Over the past 10 years, AAS has had great success in incorporating cutting-edge computerized information solutions into its day-to-day operations. The move to computerized patient charting is no different from the organization's experience in changing over to computerized dispatch and patient billing.

Currently, the deployment of the new navigator and its integration with the computerized PCDS EMS ChartWriter 2000 (CW2K) is progressing well. The related quality assurance module to accompany CW2K is nearly complete. The QI software will automatically flag run reports that are outside established data thresholds for further review beyond routine screening. Additionally, the QI system will aid the quality assurance director with descriptive statistics and data aggregation for reporting on each aspect of patient care. EMS procedures should be better quantified and reported than previous methods, with a minimum of lost data. The automation of basic statistical reports will allow the QI personnel to spend more time on data interpretation and less on report building.

The clinical database built with CW2K will also provide an accessible research data pool for the prehospital EMS research committee jointly established in 1995 between AAS and the University of New Mexico Division of Emergency Medicine. Both organizations were members of the committee performing the original research. Patient data currently come from the patient billing system combined with data from the dispatch system and manual data entry from the QI department. Once the CW2K QI system is in place, all the data from the component systems can be integrated into a single research database.

AAS plans to have a dial-up clinical database account on the new NT server being installed in the summer of 1997. CW2K will have useful data information modules added for the field personnel while in the field. Protocols for pediatric medication dosages and other timely information will be added to the help system within the basic charting system. The full rollout of the PCDS is planned for the summer of 1997, timed to coincide with the finalization and conversion of the current peer-to-peer office LAN on a Windows NT system with full Microsoft Backoffice integration and support.

The Future of Informatics at AAS

The fully functional LAN and CW2K system will close another chapter in the AAS long-range strategic plan, but it will not be the end of applied informatics at AAS. Plans have already begun for an automated employee evaluation system with supervisor data entry in mobile office units in the field. Computerized education software with dial-up, on-line EMS education is in the planning phase for implementation in early 1998.

Beyond the present and planned solutions, long-range plans call for the development of a wireless LAN allowing the field units to transmit data to hospitals and specialized hospital departments such as cardiac care facilities. Artificial intelligence is being explored for the feasibility of integrating expert systems into patient care and prehospital diagnostics. As conceived, such expert systems can be deployed via specially trained paramedics to possibly treat, then refer, patients to specialized care rather than transporting them to local emergency units. It is believed that the use of expert systems combined with established computer data collection and dispatching will allow AAS to offer primary patient care at less cost to the patient and health maintenance organizations than the treat and transport systems of today. Furthermore, this new utilization of higher trained personnel, combined with expert informatics would be a timely response to predicted rises both in the elderly population and in health care costs.

AAS is one company that is using information technology to provide quality patient care while remaining fiscally responsible. To date, the use of information technologies has allowed AAS to enjoy steady growth and advancement in the community, expanding services to meet the growth of the area with a vast array of internal improvements and advancements, all without a rate increase to the customer since 1989. A record of performance such as that would be difficult to meet in any industry, and especially in the health care field.

References

1. Eisenberg M, et al. Paramedic programs and out-of-hospital cardiac arrest. Factors associated with successful resuscitation. *Am J Public Health* 1979;69:30–38.
2. Eisenberg M, et al. Management of out-of-hospital cardiac arrest. Failure of basic emergency medical services. *JAMA* 1980;243:1049.
3. Eisenberg M, et al. Out-of-hospital cardiac arrest: Improved survival with paramedic services. *LANCET* 1980;1:812.

4. Gibson G. Measures of emergency ambulance effectiveness: Unmet need and inappropriate use. *JACEP* 1977;6:389.
5. Luterman A, et al. Evaluation of prehospital emergency medical service (EMS): Defining areas for improvement. J Trauma 1983;23:702.
6. Nagel EL. Improving emergency medical care. *N Engl J Med* 1980;302:1416.
7. National Academy of Science, National Research Council. Accidental Death and Disability: The neglected disease of modern society. Washington, DC: U.S. Department of Health, Education and Welfare; 1966.
8. Page JO, et al. Twenty years later. *JEMS* 1988;30–43.
9. Pantridge JF, JS Geddes. A Mobile Intensive care unit in the management of myocardial infarction. Lancet 1967;2:271–273.
10. Stewart RE. The training of Paramedical personnel. *Br J Anaesth* 1977;49:651–658.
11. Stout JL. Measuring your system. *JEMS* 1983;Jan:84–91.
12. Stout JL. Ambulance System Designs. *JEMS* 1986;Jan:85–99.
13. Micheal TAD. Mouth-to-lung airway for cadiac resuscitation. *Lancet* 1968;2:1329.
14. Gordon AS. The tongue-jaw lift for EOA and EGTA. *Emergency* 1981;13:40.
15. Bass R, Allison E, Hunt R. The esophageal obturator airway: A reassessment of use by paramedics. *Ann Emerg Med* 1982;11:358.
16. Donen N, et al. The esophageal obturator airway: An appraisal. *Can Anaesth Soc* 1983;30:194.
17. Micheal TAD. Comparison of the esophageal obturator airway and endotracheal intubation in prehospital ventilation during CPR. *Chest* 1985;87:814.
18. Goldenburg IF, et al. Morbidity and mortality of patients receiving the esophageal obturator airway and the endotracheal tube in prehospital cardiopulmonary arrest. *Minn Med* 1986;69:707.
19. Pepe PE, Copass MK, Joyce TH. Prehospital endotracheal intubation: Rationale for training emergency medical personnel. *Ann Emerg Med* 1985;14:1085.
20. Stewart RD, et al. Field endotracheal intubation by paramedical personnel: Success rates and complications. *Chest* 1984;85:341.
21. Stout JL. System Status Management. *JEMS* 1983;22–30.

3
Vehicle Crash Investigation

DIETMAR OTTE

In recent years in different industrial countries (e.g., the United States, Germany, France, United Kingdom, and Sweden), crash research studies were performed to identify dangerous crash situations, driver errors, and causal factors in an effort to formulate effective crash countermeasures. Most of these studies were carried out from technical, biomechanical, and/ or medical perspectives.

Vehicle crash investigations can be described as activities by manufacturers, governmental bodies, universities, or private institutes that use crash data sampling, crash reconstruction, crash simulations, and biomechanics in technical, medical, or psychological studies. Figure 3.1 describes the global structure of vehicle crash investigation.

Crash Data and Safety Milestones

Even though traffic volume worldwide continues to rise, collisions involving death or serious injuries show a generally downward trend, according to the latest edition of *World Road Statistics*, published by the International Road Federation,[1] which compiles annual statistics from 115 countries.

Since 1990, an International Road Traffic and Accident Database (IRTAD) has existed. It classifies crash data reported by the police into 240 variables.[2]

Crash statistics indicate that one of the most consistent improvements in safety rates has occurred in the area represented by the European Union.[3] This is also one of the regions of the world where road standards are most advanced and high speed motorway networks are also well developed.

Global crash statistics shown that approximately 400,000 people die annually in traffic crashes. In some countries, the decline in road injuries has been spectacular. Overall traffic volume in Western Europe has increased by about 16% over the period from 1987 to 1992. In Germany, for example,

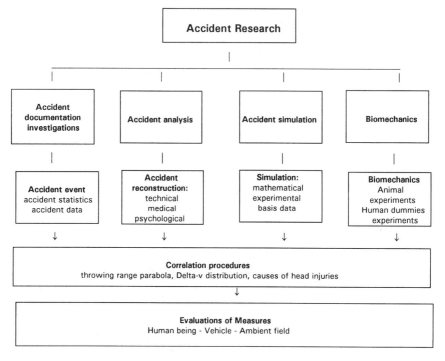

FIGURE 3.1. Structure of Accident Research.

which has the highest volume of traffic in Europe, injury and mortality rates declined steadily over the period from 1988 to 1991. In all countries, the number of fatalities on roads within towns declined from the 1970s to the 1990s (Fig. 3.2). The number of casualities from traffic crashes in the United States has declined every year since 1988. In Germany, the fatality rate within towns declined from 13.9% per 100,000 inhabitants to 3.35% per 100,000 inhabitants during the last 20 years. In the Netherlands, another country with a high volume of traffic, a fatality risk of 3.0% was recorded in today's traffic. Sweden is the country with the lowest rate of accidents on city streets. Improvement can also be measured by other statistics. For example, 30 years ago almost every second crash caused injury; today the risk is reduced to every fifth. This clearly is proof of the effectiveness of safety standards.

This reduced mortality rate is evident for all participants. Car occupants represent a predominant proportion of injured persons, as well as fatalities. In Germany, 58% of the fatally injured are car occupants, 16% are pedestrians, and 10% are cyclists.[3] This increase in safety is the result of both traffic safety initiatives and improvements in emergency care (Fig. 3.3).

Safety Measures

Rescue Service

In recent years, Emergency Medical Services (EMS) have expanded extensively in Germany. Rescue headquarters, rescue observation centers, ambulances, and rescue helicopters, as well as emergency call boxes on major

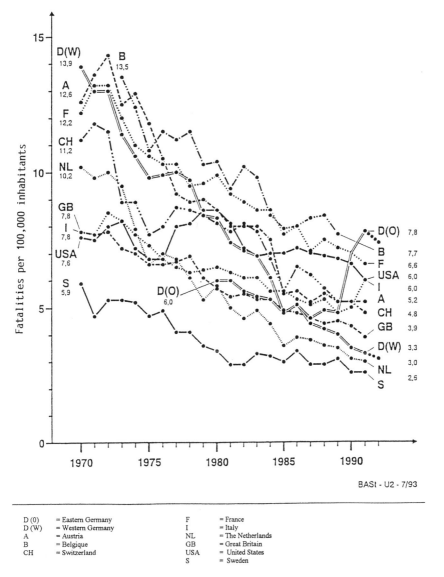

BASt - U2 - 7/93

D (0)	= Eastern Germany	F	= France
D (W)	= Western Germany	I	= Italy
A	= Austria	NL	= The Netherlands
B	= Belgique	GB	= Great Britain
CH	= Switzerland	USA	= United States
		S	= Sweden

Figure 3.2. Casualities by traffic accidents within towns per 100,000 inhabitants.

	rescue	mot two-wheelers	cars	trucks	others
1969			07/69 ECE 12 steering system		
1970	1st helicopter München		04/70 ECE 14 belt anchorage		
1972	4th helicopter Hannover	06/72 ECE 22 helmet regulation			
1973	NAW - Gummers-bacher Modell				
1974	new rescue system (call 110)		requirements belts in cars	06/74 ECE 29 interior protection	
1975			07/75 ECE 32/33 regulation car body in frontal collision		
1976		01/76 helmet using law motorcyclists	01/76 belt using law front seats		traffic safety commision police
1978		07/78 helmet using law small bikes			
1980	model NEF/NAW Unterfranken integrated medical doctor	04/80 driving school chances	06/80 ECE 42 bumper recommendations		
1981			02/81 ECE 43 safety glass 02/81 ECE 44 child restraint systems		
1983	80% covering area helicopters (34)			07/83 ECE 58 underdriving protection	
1984	100% covering area helicopters (35)		08/74 fine for nonusing front seat belts 08/74 belt using law rear seats		
1985		10/85 helmet using law moped riders			03/85 30 km/h-areas
1986			01/86 fine for nonusing rear seat belts	12/86 ECE 66 compartment stiffness bus	
1988				01/88 ECE 73 side protection	
1991				10/91 ABS	
1992				01/92 side protection new trucks >3,5t	
1993			04/93 use law for child restraint systems		
1994			06/94 partial std. airbag equipment	01/94 side protection all trucks >3,5t	

FIGURE 3.3. Regulations by government for traffic safety (01/76 means month/year).

highways and motorways have been established. For example, in 1970, at the time of the highest fatality rate, the first rescue helicopter was stationed in Munich. By 1983, 80% of the country was covered by air medical capability. In 1984, this reached 100%. The establishment of a standardized emergency telephone system for police and fire services was completed in 1984. Research regarding the rescue system is conducted by the Federal Institute of Transport, the Federal Highway Institute, and the Federal Ministry of Research and Technology.

In the United States, trauma centers were established. Special attention to quality of care followed. However, the time lapse for qualified help to reach the injured remains, as before, an important factor in improving outcome in any rescue system. For 10 years, more than 90% of emergency patients were treated within 10 minutes after the alarm was raised by the rescue service. In the future, more attention must be paid to the process of vehicle crash rescue and extrication of victims.

Vehicle Safety

Safety devices, such as seat belts, child restraint systems, and front and side protections on cars, have become widespread in recent years. In accordance with the guidelines of the U.S. Federal Motor Vehicle Safety Standards (FMVSS), the European Union (EU) and the Economic Commission for Europe (ECE), manufacturers must adhere to optimal safety standards for vehicle passengers and external traffic participants, such as pedestrians and cyclists.

The car design and construction must now pass through multiple phases of development, including continuous changes in the vehicle's exterior and interior geometry. Further refinements have occurred in the design of front and side structures, integrated energy absorbing steering wheels, safety belts, and airbags.

Accident Simulations and Data Analysis

The advances in traffic safety, especially from the vehicular standpoint, are based mainly on the results of crash tests and biomechanical simulations with humanlike bodies, so-called "crash test dummies." Tests with human bodies, called "postmortal test objects" (PMTO) or human dummies (HD), also contribute to an improved understanding of crash dynamics.

In the 1970s, investigations by Patrick[4] disclosed that injury severity for vehicle occupants was influenced by deceleration during the collision and the period of time of the deceleration. High-speed changes over long distances and time lapses did not appear to lead to injuries, but falls from low heights or low-speed changes that occurred over a very short time interval did have fatal consequences. This phenomenon was well known to the aircraft industry, which was the first to test for definition of the endurance limit. Tests had begun in the 1950s, conducted by the U.S. Air Force. Stapp applied these observations to the area of vehicle safety and recommended a continuous exchange of experiences across descriptives.[5] Since 1954, the annual so-called STAPP Car Crash Conference in the United States has served to promote the exchange of biomechanical information. Speed, deceleration, and time of deceleration are established physical measures. The resultant injury and injury severity are often missing. Therefore, human tolerance values are necessary for this definition.

In the 1970s, a world-wide network of institutions carried out crash analyses and experimental work with crash test dummies. Such tests were first conducted only in the U.S. and France; in Germany, mainly forensic work was reported. Tests with living persons yield limited results, because many protective measures must be taken to protect the test persons, only low speeds are permissible, and all injuries must be avoided. For this reason, estimation of biomechanical limitations based on tests with subjects is restricted. Patrick[4] demonstrated that the tolerance level for slight injuries of the thorax is 60 g. For test subjects, this must be limited to 20 g. When the results are tabulated to reflect anatomic differences by age and sex, considerable differences are revealed and the resulting injuries depend on impact point, geometry, and impact direction. For these reasons, substitutes were sought for live subjects. One of the best-documented tolerance values originated from the Air Force ejector seat, which is constructed to create a 20 g deceleration without injuries. Based on tests with volunteers and bodies, the tolerance time limit for head injuries was determined. An extensive measuring series with bodies at Wayne State University in Detroit led to the so-called Wayne State University Curve, which is the basis of various improvements in vehicle safety. Based on results with living subjects and cadavers, norms were compiled. The maximum of head deceleration could be defined as 80 g with an injury criterion of less than 3 ms.[7] Today, advances in road traffic and vehicle development are measured against this 80 g criterion. Further capacity criteria are still being defined, including head injury criteria (HIC) and other parameters for thorax, thigh, and knee impact. Current results of crash analyses, crash tests, and tests on cadavers supply much needed data for improved vehicle safety. Crash data are essential for ongoing validation.

For this reason, extensive accident analyses are carried out, in which injuries are documented and scientifically processed. A worldwide network of in-depth crash investigations was established to describe injuries occurring from real crashes and under certain crash conditions. In America, the National Accident Sampling Systems (NASS) was established in 1970, with 30 teams of engineers and doctors collecting accident data.[6] In many European countries too, research centers were established. The French Organisme National de Securité Routière (ONSER) is one example. In Germany, the Federal Highway Research Institute (BASt) collects data from investigations conducted at accident sites by the Accident Research Unit (ARU) of the Medical University of Hannover.[8]

Importance of Existing Car Safety Concepts for the Accident Safety Level

This section attempts to quantify the effectiveness of safety devices in cars that are responsible for the reduction in vehicular fatalities. This analysis compares accident data from old and newer vehicles. The accident data analysis of the ARU at the Medical University Hannover is the basis for this report.

For comparison, crashes from 1985 until 1990 were evaluated and compared with data on cars manufactured up to 1980, described as "old vehicles," versus those manufactured since 1981, described as "new vehicles." To keep the number of influential variables for crashes with personal injury as low as possible, only drivers involved in isolated frontal collision (i.e., no multiple collisions), and passengers involved in lateral collisions, who had been sitting on the impact side (i.e., not those on the opposite side) were analyzed. Vehicle weight was differentiated by a curb weight of up to 1000 kilos (described as "light cars"), and more than 1000 kilos (described as "heavy cars"). The injuries were documented in detail and classified in correlation with the Abbreviated Injury Scale (AIS).[9]

The most frequent collision type resulting in injured persons, excluding pedestrians and cyclists, is the frontal impact, by approximately 60% of the cases. Lateral collisions were registered at approximately 27% of cars, and rear collisions at 13% of the cases (Fig. 3.4).

This distribution by collision types shows that today's car passengers are more often injured in lateral collisions. As a result of seatbelt effectiveness, the number of injuries resulting from frontal collisions has been continuously reduced during the past years to 54%, while injuries from lateral collisions have seen a relative increase to 27% (Fig. 3.5).

Full overlapping of frontal and side impacts is rare. As a rule, the vehicles may be partly overlapping, mostly between one-third and two-thirds of the front in eccentric impact situations. In lateral collisions, the passenger side of the vehicle is often involved.

Frontal Collisions

The protective effect of the seatbelt was established for old as well as for new vehicles. The injury severity for nonbelt-protected drivers, for instance, shows a rather progressive increase, with rising speed absorption (delta-v).

Delta-v, which describes the severity of an accident as a result of the speed change within the collision, represents the load on the passengers.

Collision Types of 1384 cars, Manufacturing year since 1980
single collisions only (without pedestrians and two-wheelers)

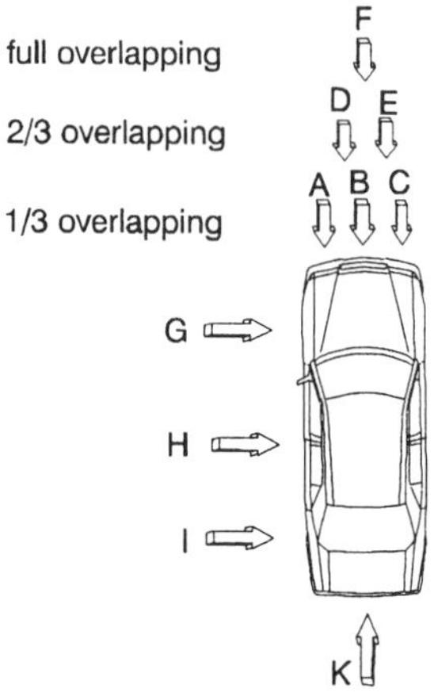

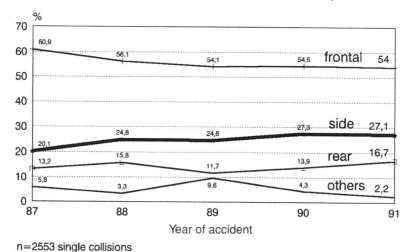

		frequen-cies	uninjured	MAIS 1/2	MAIS 3/4	MAIS 5/6
frontal	A	8,7	54,7	90,7	9,3	-
	B	2,9	24,1	86,46	9,1	4,5
	C	4,6	55,8	100	-	-
	D	8,9	41,4	84,5	13,8	1,7
	E	8,3	48,9	80,4	15,2	4,3
	F	26,1	37,8	87,4	9,3	3,3
side	G	7,7	47,6	97,7	2,3	-
	H	17,8	23,9	78,3	11,2	10,5
	I	2,3	54,5	100	-	-
rear	K	12,6	43,2	100	-	-
	total	100	40,4	87,6	8,6	3,9

full overlapping

2/3 overlapping

1/3 overlapping

Accident Research Unit Hannover

FIGURE 3.4. Frequency and injury severity for different collision types.

Impact Situation of Cars
(without coll. with pedestrians/two-wheelers)

n=2553 single collisions

FIGURE 3.5. Frequency of side impacts in car collisions in relation to other kinds of impacts.

549 drivers without seat-belt

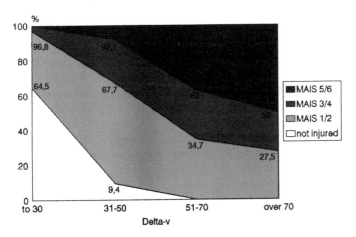

296 drivers with seat-belt

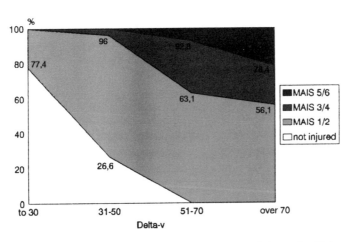

FIGURE 3.6. Injury severity MAIS and Delta-*v* for cars with frontal collision, manufacturing years to 1980, and curb weight up to 1000 kg.

Delta-*v* is evaluated with the mathematical reconstruction calculation and differs from energy equivalent speed (EES), which represents the deformation pattern. A higher injury threshold is evident in all Delta-*v* levels for heavier vehicles rather than for lighter vehicles.

Figure 3.6 compares belted and nonbelted situations and Figure 3.7 plots the differences in severity of injury between drivers of light and heavy cars. Without a belt in car weights less than 1000 kg and Delta-*v* values up to

523 drivers, cars to 1000 kg

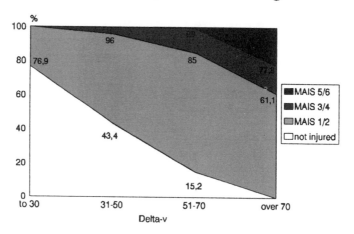

374 drivers, cars over 1000 kg

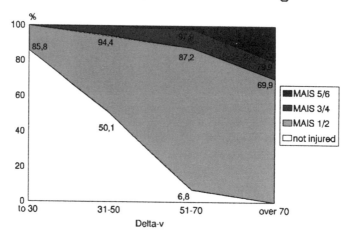

FIGURE 3.7. Injury severity MAIS of drivers wearing seatbelts and Delta-*v* for cars with frontal collision, manufacturing years from 1981.

30 km/h, 64.5% of the drivers remained without injury, 3.2% suffered injury severity rated at MAIS 5/6 (maximum AIS) or greater. In Delta-*v* values from 51 to 70 km/h, all sustained injury, 34.7% suffering MAIS 1/2, and 37% MAIS 5/6. In heavier vehicles, however, more uninjured persons were registered for all Delta-*v* values, especially up to 30 km/h (85.8%), and at 51 to 70 km/h (still only 24%). Even when belts are used, however, lighter vehicles have significantly more severely injured drivers (MAIS 5/6) compared to heavy vehicles. Thus, belt usage results in a reduction in injuries in both light and heavy vehicles.

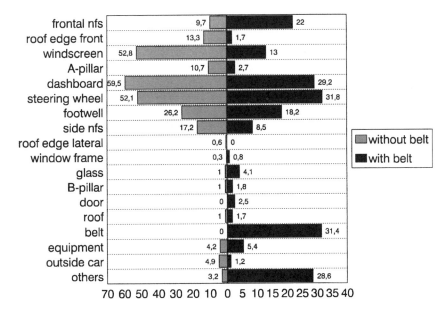

FIGURE 3.8. Parts causing injury to drivers in frontal collisions, manufacturing years to 1980 and curb weight up to 1000 kg.

The injury sources inside the vehicle have also changed because of the belt usage (Fig. 3.8). For the nonbelted drivers, the parts that most frequently caused injuries were the steering wheel, the dashboard, and the windshield. These are less common sources of injury for drivers who wore seatbelts. With belt usage in particular, the windshield is very rarely involved. This is almost equally true with light as well as heavy cars. For heavier vehicles, a lower injury frequency is also evident. In car weights up to 1000 kg and manufactured up to 1980, nonbelted drivers were injured by the steering wheel in 59.5% of cases, and belted persons in 31.8%. In cars weighing more than 1000 kg, drivers without belts were injured in 52.1% of cases, versus only 19.4% for those using belts.

Injuries caused by the footwell area, however, are reduced only minimally with belt usage. This means that even when seatbelts are worn, the footwell is one of the main sources of injury in the vehicle interior. There are no visible changes in the injury situation between old and newer vehicles. In both, 18% of the drivers were injured by parts of the footwell.

Lateral Collisions

The protective effect of the seatbelt is not comprehensive in lateral collisions because laterally, a crumple zone region is missing (Fig. 3.9). Further,

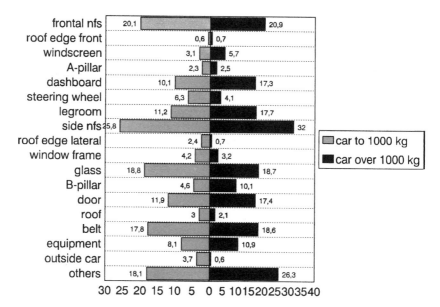

Figure 3.9. Parts causing injury to passengers wearing seatbelts at side impact, front seated on impact side.

because the passenger in the seat on the impact side is moving relatively in the direction of the impact region, he or she is exposed to deforming interior structures. For light as well as for heavy vehicles, an almost similar increase in injury severity is observed, with increasing speed and Delta-v. At up to 30 km/h, 56% of the impact-nearside sitting passengers are injured in light as well as in heavier vehicles. In lighter vehicles with Delta-v values of 31 to 50 km/h, 12.8% of the passengers were not injured; in heavy vehicles, however, the statistic remains 21%.

Fifty-one percent of the drivers in cars with weights of 1000 kg and 59.8% in vehicles with weights of more than 1000 kg suffered injuries from lateral structures (Fig. 3.9). At first, the low number of injury-causing side parts appears remarkable. The reason is the resulting relative movement of the passengers, which is determined by the impulse angle and is caused by the collision mode and speed vectors of the colliding vehicles. In an oblique collision, an oblique relative movement of the passengers is often caused by the rotation of the vehicle. The passengers impact with the interior front parts. In heavy vehicles, a more frequent source of injury is established at lateral B-pillars. In cars above 1000 kg, 10.1% of the passengers are injured by these parts, in comparison with 4.6% in light cars.

In lateral collisions, injuries from impact with the dashboard are possible in more than 10.1% of cases in light vehicles and 17.3% in heavy vehicles. The steering wheel must also be regarded as an injury source in 4 to 6% of lateral collisions, with the steering wheel and the A-pillar causing especially serious injuries (approximately 40 to 50% AIS 1). In lateral collisions, impact situations with relatively sharp parts of the side region, such as the roof edge, B-pillar, and window frame, caused serious injuries more frequently in heavier vehicles.

The injury severity in side collisions is influenced considerably by the degree of intrusion. Often the front part of the impacting vehicle penetrates the side region (i.e., the region of the front A-pillar that leads to deformations) which causes a restriction in the survival space for the occupants.

Pedestrian Collisions

When a car collides with a pedestrian, the leg region will be pushed away and consequently, the pedestrian will impact with the front hood of the car. Depending on the impact speed, the victim may be pushed forward to the windshield. Significant injuries are caused by the impact of the pedestrian's lower legs with the bumper, knee and thigh region with the edges of the front hood, and head with the front hood or the windshield.

The differention of vehicles by the manufacturing year (i.e., before and after 1980) shows that for all body regions of injured pedestrians, with the exception of the thorax, a lower number of injuries was registered for newer vehicles. In collisions with vehicles manufactured after 1980, 57.4% of the pedestrians suffered head injuries, compared with 64.2% in collisions with vehicles manufactured before 1980. Only thorax injuries were more frequent, with 25.5% for newer vehicles, compared with old vehicles. Basically, with the exception of neck and abdominal injuries, newer vehicles registered a slightly greater number of injuries. The reason is that more newer vehicles are built as compacts, with a short-length front hood. For leg injuries, there are no apparent differences between older and newer vehicles. As far as the distribution of the injury severity degree for the legs is concerned, no significant differences could be observed between standard protruding bumpers and the integrated bumpers in newer vehicles. With the integrated bumpers, fewer complex fractures of the tibia occur. The third-degree open fractures that often involve long-term consequences are quite rare. Because of the flat-faced bumper form, the impact force is transferred broadly. With the integrated bumper, on the other hand, ankle joint and knee instabilities may be more frequent, as a result of the great bending effect for the foot and leg region. The expected decrease in injury severity for pedestrians because of the modification of the front shape of vehicles is, therefore, not apparent in comparisons between old and new vehicles. With newer vehicles, in similar collision speeds, pedestrians are more frequently seriously injured (Fig. 3.10). A cause may be the light vehicles with compact construction and short front hood length, in which the upper body, including the head, hits the front hood or its frame structure, respectively, at lower collision speeds.

manufacturing year of car to 1980

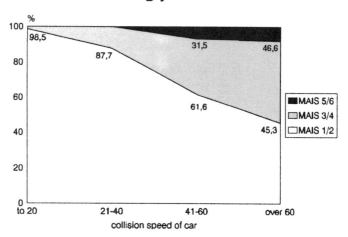

collision speed of car

manufacturing year of car after 1980

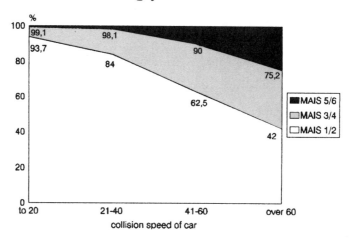

collision speed of car

FIGURE 3.10. Injury Severity MAIS of pedestrians and collision speed of cars in single frontal collisions.

State of Affairs in Passenger Safety

This study showed that the safety of a car is based on the different safety devices and on the weight of the car. Passengers in heavy vehicles in today's crashes are subjected to less severe injuries. Particularly in lateral collisions, the weight of the impacting vehicle influences the severity of the injury. When the impacting vehicle is heavier than the impacted one, the injury risk is very much higher. As a rule, heavier vehicles have longer frontal deformation zones and delta-v is lower. In the future, measures should be taken to ensure that if the striking vehicle is heavier, it should absorb the main portion of the resulting impact energy. This means that optimized development of the vehicle front would lead to improvement in lateral safety.

The seatbelt has changed injury patterns in a very positive direction. Injury frequency, as well as severity, were reduced by belt usage. But in many cars, parts of the car interior (i.e., dashboard and steering wheel) are a source of injuries in frontal impacts. For this reason, the footwell must still be regarded as a main injury source, even with belt usage. Further advances in safety are needed in this region.

Foot fractures are injuries with serious consequences.[10] Ankle and foot injuries demand the longest stationary treatment (18%), have the highest complication rate (19%), and require the highest rate of rehabilitation (21%). A calcaneus fracture often results in permanent disability, with a reduced working ability of 25%. A fracture of the ankle joint causes a functional loss of 26%. From a traumatological point of view, this justifies demands for improved design of the footwell area. Such improvements could include:

- stable passenger compartment in the foot room region, inclusive side structure, and the drive shaft tunnel;
- padding of the floor to reduce the impact force;
- protective shaping of the pedal region to reduce the injury by increasing the effect of the axial load and the rotation movement of the foot;
- modification of the dashboard by padding; and
- more moving space above the foot room region.

In view of these facts, efforts by car manufacturers to reduce injury occurrence, especially to the head, would benefit from a pulling-away device for the steering wheel (procon-ten) or the installation of an airbag. In actual crashes, however, it was shown that the effectiveness of procon-ten was limited. A frontal impact, with the inclusion of the engine block in almost longitudinal direction, is quite rare. An airbag seems to be more effective. The downward moving head is slowed down and experiences a load reduction by the airbag.

The effectiveness of the airbag on Germany's roads has not been quantified, because few vehicles have been equipped with it. However, ARU Hannover's critical evaluation of accident data shows that the maximum effectiveness of the airbag as quantified by computer modeling. The result is that the severity degree MAIS 6 could be totally eliminated by the airbag. Fifty-six percent of the serious injuries (MAIS 4–6), 30% of serious (MAIS 2–3) as well as 13% of slight injuries (MAIS 1) would be avoidable. The proportion of uninjured persons would increase by 11%.

These conclusions resulted from a computer determination that eliminated all injuries avoided by airbag deployment under frontal impact to an angle of +30 degrees. These were:

- injuries by head impact with the steering wheel, the windshield, and the A-pillar of the dashboard;
- thoracic injuries caused by pressure from the seatbelt or strong chest impacts with the steering wheel; and
- injuries caused by impact of the abdomen with the steering wheel.

The calculation is based on a statistical weighting procedure of the documented accidents in the ARU.

Measures for increased safety in lateral collisions must include the side structures. An airbag for lateral protection seems to be an efficient construction. The evaluation of investigations of accidents would recommend that this airbag cover the upper part of the door to reduce the contact with glass and frames. Standardized crash tests would help to produce an improved safety level for all vehicles. But they could also increase the dissimilarity of the safety level between light and heavy vehicles. They have to be carried out with consideration of the possible disparity in vehicle size. The installation of the airbag should not only fulfill the test criteria, but the safety gain should be profitable.

Crash test conditions have to be adapted to real crash situations. For frontal collisions, a 40% offset impact to the front is the best test condition in terms of conforming to reality. For lateral collisions, test conditions should be in an oblique direction, between 30 and 45 degrees frontally. Impact, conforming to reality, should be slightly in front of the center of gravity with a Delta-v value of 40 km/h. The height of the impacting barrier should be more than 300 mm. On the dummy, besides evaluating head and thorax injuries, the load on the foot and tibia should be measured with different forces and moments.

Data show that the newer exterior shaping of the car did not reduce the injury severity of pedestrians in the expected manner. Accident statistics for pedestrians demonstrate that a continuous reduction in the number of fatally injured persons could be observed. The positive measures for shaping the car exterior were negated by the compact design, with its short fronthood length. The established increased injury risk with short fronthoods is not based on the fronthood itself, but on more frequent windshield impacts at lower speeds. Short fronthoods appear to be more sensible, if the adjoining glass region is also modified. An integrated line of fronthood and windshield, with a pronounced inclination, appears to be preferable. The continuous reduction of fatalities is related to the reduced collision speeds in local traffic. An analysis of the collision speed range revealed that 21% of all car drivers on city roads exceeded the permissible speed of 50 km/h. On city roads, 28% of accidents could be avoided if the drivers obeyed posted speed regulations.

Clearly, the reduction in the number of traffic fatalities is mainly the result of measures taken to increase vehicle safety. The most important are passive safety devices. Despite the decreasing injury risk and severity risk in crashes, the number of crashes continues to increase because of more and more vehicle registrations. Therefore measures for crash avoidance have to be part of prevention strategies. The safety standard is, however, different from car to car and is influenced by the size of the vehicle, by the vehicle's mass, by the installed safety devices, and by the attitudes of the designer and the driver. Beyond this, a minimum standard is dictated by law, which in individual crash situations assures a certain safety. Vehicle safety and driving regulations are revised from year to year, as a result of research, public pressure, and the attitudes of car manufacturers. The severity of an injury in a crash is a result of a physical process, i.e., transformation of energy, the kinematics of vehicle occupants, and human tolerance. Injuries are the result of different variables, such as impact modes between large and small vehicles, point of impact on the car related to stiff and soft regions, and the effectiveness of safety devices.

Further injury reduction in Germany could be achieved by limiting speed. This was determined by the computer modeling at ARU Hannover, which made the following observations.

1. On city roads, driving speed should be limited to 50 km/h. This would result in the prevention of 28% of fatal crashes, 7% of severe injury producing crashes, and 5% of minor crashes.
2. On rural roads, driving speed should be adapted to the situation, i.e., driving not more than 80 km/h would result in prevention of 8% of fatal crashes, 9% of severe crashes, and 6% of minor crashes.
3. On highways, however, injury and crash prevention seem not to be affected by speed limitation.

Regulation of vehicular speed is a main point in safety prevention measures. It relates to discussions about heavy traffic, ecologic strain, and alternative traffic concepts, which were initiated by the increase of street traffic and infrastructure limitations. The ideal circumstance would take traffic out of towns, with the construction of smaller vehicles for town regions. Traffic separation measures, such as the separation of motorized and nonmotorized traffic, as well as speed-reducing measures, therefore, have a considerable influence on the resulting crash pattern and statistics.

Injury prevention is a multifunctional task that requires cooperation among manufacturers, governments, and researchers on questions of biomechanics, vehicle crashworthiness and crash prevention, and analysis of data.

The Role of Accident Statistics

Existing in-depth studies vary widely in their objectives, philosophy, methodology, modeling, data collection, and data analysis. They are designed to describe, in part or as a whole, the multicausal events of a crash—the interacting factors and mechanisms. A special feature is to describe injury patterns in correlation to their causing factors. Some studies focus on the traffic process altogether, others on the interactions of the various elements (e.g., road user and vehicle environment), and still others on the role of the driver. The aim of all special investigators is to create a database with more and better crash data than is otherwise available from official statistics that are based on police reports, which are also known as national accident statistics.

In principle, two basic data levels are useful.

Data of the official traffic crash statistics. Crashes involving injured persons and crashes leading to property damage above a certain level are documented by police reports and are available in a national database. This data source exists in every country. These data are compressed together in IRTAD, the International Road Traffic and Accident Database.

Data from crash investigations at the site of the crash. In some countries, investigations are simulating the actual crash. The main investigators are:

USA   National Accident Safety System (NASS)
France   INRETS
UK   RICE University of Loughbourogh
Germany   ARU Medical University Hannover

Both data levels are necessary to answer questions concerning traffic safety.

In-depth road crash investigations can provide more profound and detailed knowledge about different factors causing crashes and their consequences than can the records based on routine police investigations, hospital registrations, or insurance claims. The explanation is obvious. These forms and records are primarily intended to serve other objectives. The reason for studying the crash mechanisms is equally obvious. In many respects, what ordinary records can offer as a basis for integrated road safety programs have already been shown to be ineffective.

Crash data is best distinguished by the different crash phases described as follows: Precrash is the interaction between road user, vehicle, and the road and traffic environment. Crash is the collection of external and internal environmental factors, such as vehicle design, and the effect of safety systems. Postcrash is the vehicle crash rescue, including emergency medical services, trauma care, and rehabilitation. It is essential that the general approach or underlying philosophy of an in-depth study is articulated. The approach may be of the kind in which in-depth investigations, laboratory experiments, and theoretical model simulations are combined.

The collection of crash data from all phases provides information concerning the crash outcome. Because a crash is the result of the interaction among humans, vehicles, and environments, measures taken toward crash and injury prevention must focus on these three factors. This means that there are different users of this information, including the car industry, the insurance associations, and legislators. The information can be characterized by the human factor, the vehicle design, and environmental factors.

The investigation of crashes differentiates between measures taken toward the reduction of injury consequences (passive safety) and the prevention of crashes (active safety). Information correlating injury and vehicle deformation are more important for reducing injury severity, whereas aspects of driver behaviors and the precrash events are of central importance for crash avoidance. In most settings, different disciplines are involved at different levels. The individuals most concerned with in-depth investigations are engineers, surgeons, psychologists, and statisticians.

In-depth investigations have been performed for different purposes, using different methods preferred by various interest groups. The approach of the investigation is determined by the purpose of the study. Police files are the starting point for most in-depth investigations. Police crash statistics, which have already been documented, may be further analyzed by a scientific team, according to its own areas of interest. Information from hospitals, patients, and vehicle inspections is also collected. In the Hannover region of Germany, the teams often drive directly to the crash scene immediately after it has occurred, on condition that the team is integrated into the information systems of the police and rescue services (example: ARU Hannover/Germany).

Many of these investigations have either been discontinued or are of limited scope. But some of them have continued and resulted in important crash research on a national level. They can be divided into three different kinds of sponsorships: those financed by the government (e.g. Germany and the United States); those financed by a combination of the government and the car industry (e.g., France and the United Kingdom); and those financed by the car industry (e.g., Sweden).

In countries in which the government is the only financer, the car industry usually finances its own in-depth investigations (e.g., Mercedes and BMW in Germany).

Early arrival at the crash scene increases the possibilities for accurately describing the characteristics of the crash.

On scene: Investigation starts at the scene of the crash, immediately after the crash with the vehicle(s) still in place.

On site: Investigation includes only a documentation of characteristics of the crash site. A time definition for the crash is not given.

Retrospective: Investigation is based on written reports, without observation of crash site.

For questions concerning crashes that occurred under the influence of alcohol, day and night times have to be taken into consideration. The time of crash occurrence is important for these questions. The possibility of documentation of crash characteristics depends on the study design.

Braking traces, for instance, can only be described if they are investigated and photographed at the crash site or evaluated by experts. The pattern of specific injuries can only be described after observing and analyzing victims. The place of investigation, as well as the time of documentation, are of special importance in regard to these questions.

The reliability of immediate on-scene or retrospective data relates to exactness and quality of the investigation. Documentation carried out by a team of specialists, in accordance with its own scientific criteria, opens up the possibility for major advances in future crash prevention.

References

1. IRF. World Road Statistics 1988–1992. Geneva: International Road Federation; 1993.
2. Brühning E, Berns S. IRTAD. International Road Traffic and Accident Database. *Zeitschrift Verkehrssicherheit* 1993;39:121–124.
3. StBA: Verkehrsunfälle in der Bundesrepublik Deutschland Statistisches Bundesamt Wiesbaden, Fachserie 8, Reihe 7. Verlag Metzler-Poeschel; 1993.
4. Patrick LM. Human tolerance to impact and its application to safety design. Proc. 19th Stapp Car Crash Conference; 1975.
5. Stapp JP. Review of Air Force research on biodynamics of collision injury. Proc. 10th Stapp Car Crash Conference; 1966.
6. Nahum AM, Gatts JD, Gadd GW, Danforth J. Impact tolerance of the skull and face. Proc. 12th Stapp Car Crash Conference; 1968.
7. Nash CE, McDonald S. New technologies and techniques for NASS accident investigations. Detroit, 1985.
8. Otte D. The Accident Research Unit Hannover as example for importance and benefit of existing in depth investigations. Proc. International Congress & Exposition; Detroit; 1994.
9. The Abbreviated Injury Scale, Revision 90. American Association for Automotive Medicine; 1985.
10. Berufsgenossenschaften e.V. Verletzungsfolgen nach Straßenverkehrsunfällen Schriftenreihe des Hauptverbandes der gewerblichen. Siegburg: Berufsgenossenschaften; 1990.

4
Informatics in the Emergency Department

Mark C. Henry, Lester Kallus, Peter Viccellio, and Todd B. Taylor

It is 3 A.M. at the local hospital. Three victims from a motor vehicle collision are en route to the emergency department. Vital signs and pertinent prehospital findings have already been transmitted. You look at the patient flow screen to see the current census and open rooms.

The three patients arrive nearly simultaneously. All pertinent admission information is instantly obtained via magnetic card. When the patients arrive in the treatment area, charts have been printed.

Patient 1 has a laceration. Electronic images pre- and postrepair are captured and stored on the patient database. The patient's tetanus history is obtained from his magnetic card. An appointment is automatically made for wound check and suture removal. The patient is placed on pain medication. Customized discharge instructions and drug information are automatically generated. The use of a suture tray and two packs of 4-0 nylon has been recorded on the patient's bill. This entry, in turn, automatically notifies Central Sterile to replace the depleted supplies.

Patient 2, a restrained passenger with a chest abrasion from the seat belt, has mild chest pain; chest x-ray shows a borderline widened mediastinum, and electrocardiogram reveals a right bundle branch block (RBBB). A previous x-ray at Samaritan Hospital, available via teleradiology, shows that the size of the mediastinum is unchanged. The patient's RBBB is discovered from two sources: an ECG stored in Samaritan Hospital's database and a notation on the patient's personal ID card. After appropriate monitoring, the patient is discharged for follow-up with his private physician. Today's chest film and ECG and a record of the emergent medical care are transmitted to the private physician.

Patient 3 has an open femur fracture. The magnetic history indicates:

a history of a seizure disorder managed with carbamazepine and valproic acid
an allergy to penicillin and cephalosporin drugs

To ensure that appropriate therapy is chosen, you use DRUGDEX to assist in selecting a drug. The compound recommended is ordered electronically from Pharmacy and instantly cross-indexed against carbamazepine and valproic acid. Simultaneously, the cost of the drug is added to the patient's billing record.

Patient 3 is then wheeled to the OR for wound debridement. The digital image of his fracture that is being viewed in the OR suite has already been viewed remotely by a radiologist covering five hospitals at this predawn hour. The specialist's report is seen attached to the electronic image.

Introduction

The connotations of computerized entry, storage, and display of information regarding care of trauma patients in the emergency department are vast. The intelligent application of computerized recording and transmission of patient data will result in quantum leaps in efficiency. It will help match personnel and equipment more closely to patient demands. It can network every participating emergency department with multistate studies of trauma research and injury prevention.

Educational resources such as clinical guidelines and drug reaction databanks would be incorporated automatically into care plans. Digitized images will permit practitioners in the hospital and at remote settings to share scene photographs and digitized radiographs. Discharge instructions will be individualized for each patient, and copies of individual medical records will be easily retrievable during follow-up care.

Compliance with mandated reporting requirements will be automatically fulfilled, prompted by screens on the history and physical examination, and updated as necessary in real time by laboratory results.

In specific clinical situations, MEDLINE can be searched in real time to find appropriate clinical studies relating to a patient's problem. With such backup, the physician can both provide the most current treatment and find guidance in treating uncommon or unusual clinical problems.

As a result, patient care will improve. Because of individualized instructions, the ability to easily apply appropriate clinical guidelines, and easy retrieval and transmission of clinical information, the image of the emergency department (ED) will change from a costly setting, where the norm is defensive medicine, to one of efficiency and effectiveness.

Prehospital Care

Medical Control

Once information concerning an injured patient has been obtained, automated notification can deploy the trauma team or place its members on alert. For example, pager equipment incorporating LCD screens could be used to inform the trauma team of the type and extent of trauma. Digitized images from the scene could be transmitted prior to arrival of the patient and appended to the medical record. Templates could identify transfer candidates and forward complete records prior to arrival of the victims.

Clinical Care

Triage Desk

Registration of victims of minor trauma can be accomplished with minimal nursing input. Patients or their families working at touch screens could enter demographic data and describe the chief complaint. Pulse and blood pressure would be taken automatically and entered directly into the patient's record.

Triage personnel could initiate order entry according to clinical guidelines such as the Ottawa ankle rules, thus minimizing the patient's time in the treatment area.

Computerized Record with Pen Pad at Bedside

Patient records that reside on a network will incorporate prehospital information. These data and more detailed findings communicated by paramedics during transfer of patient care to the ED staffs can be fed back to medical control to upgrade the data for future efforts in continuous quality improvement (CQI). Templates for history and physical exam results can be based in part on mechanism of injury. Treatment guidelines would assist practitioners in standardizing their care. Preset algorithms for ordering head computerized tomographic (CT) scans and blood studies would reflect local practice guidelines and might insulate the practitioner from "Monday morning quarterbacking," obviating questions about medical necessity and preauthorization.

Order entry placed by the practitioner would be immediately transmitted to appropriate departments (phlebotomy, radiology, pharmacy). The data would also be placed on the patient's bill. All medications ordered would be checked for compatibility with each other and with medications and conditions noted on the patient's medical history.

Screening for problems such as domestic violence could be suggested for a patient found to have visited several emergency departments with varying forms of minor but inadequately explained trauma.

Mode of Inscription: Voice Versus Printed Chart

Voice recognition systems, which allow for immediate transcription and thus immediate availability of a typed, legible record, are gaining popularity as the technology improves. Many emergency departments across the country have already adopted voice transcription.

In other departments, where a voice record is awaiting manual transcription, a digitized voice record can be made available so that a given verbal report can be accessed before the record has been transcribed. Similarly, a voice recording from a radiologist or consulting specialist could be reviewed immediately.

Digitized Images

Digital cameras are now available. Prices are dropping dramatically at the same time that resolution is increasing. Digitized images can help patient care in multiple areas:

Blunt trauma: a digitized image of the vehicle can be part of the record, which will help practitioners understand the mechanism of injury.

Wound management: an image of a patient's would entered into the record would replace the 35mm slide classically collected and filed by the plastic surgeon. Hospitals are already creating secure electronic recording mechanisms such as stacked laser disks. Wound images at time of wound check or suture removal would assist in gauging effectiveness of techniques in wound management.

Wound documentation: medical legal documentation of assault and family violence would be incorporated in patient records and made available to individual patients and to legal authorities.

Teleradiology: this technology is already being incorporated in institutions across the country for magnetic resonance imaging and CT scans. Patients needing a study at one hospital can have results of studies from other institutions transmitted via modem for immediate comparison. In the near future, all radiological studies will be recorded electronically. As the digitized radiological image begins to replace x-ray film, we may find radiologists reviewing x-ray data for more than one hospital without having to travel between institutions. At off-hours, one radiologist could cover several hospitals, giving instantaneous official readings of all studies. All these studies could be viewed by the practitioner at the bedside or in the operating room, on monitors. Lost films will be a thing of the past. Similarly, old films may be instantly retrieved for comparison.

Mandated Reporting

Mandated reporting can be automated so that the practitioner need only manage the patient. The reporting would be generated by the patient care system, with key fields automatically loaded based on chief complaint or mechanism of injury. Patients with carbon monoxide poisoning, serious assaults, or large burns would be automatically entered into the appropriate part of the system, which would generate the necessary forms and electronically transmit them to fulfill reporting requirements.

Discharge Instructions

Illegible discharge instructions would be replaced by individualized discharge instructions from a standard database.

Inventory and Billing

Automated billing based on extraction of information in the electronic medical record can assure accuracy and completeness in patient billing. For example, when a tray is used, billing will be automatically entered at the same time that Central Supply receives notification to send a replacement. Improved accuracy in coding will be of value for reimbursement as well as retrospective clinical studies.

Patient Tracking

As the patient is moved within the emergency department, an annotated chart could be displayed on a board, to keep everyone aware of the patient's status.

CQI and Trauma Research

Quality Assurance

Prehospital data would be double-checked by EMS personnel in the ED before returning to service. They could verify information relayed in advance by medical control, as well as complete electronic forms detailing essential historical and physical exam results, treatment, serial vital signs, and response to treatment. This information will improve Medical Control's quality review and increase the value of subsequent feedback to EMS squads and the service medical directors.

Several CQI programs are already available to individualize reports to practitioners. These CQI programs, as they become incorporated into patient records, will standardize CQI practices across wide areas.

Credentialing of residents can be automated when the record of the procedure interfaces with a program that tracks resident procedures.

Research Implications

Trauma patients discharged from the hospital after being examined and perhaps treated in the ED are not included in traditional trauma registries.

As computerized records become available with vital signs and critical scores entered, trauma registries can begin to automatically incorporate this large number of missing patients.

Current Status

No one system is capable currently of all the desirable features informatics can provide. Nevertheless, much of what has been mentioned can easily be done with available technology. We have several options. We can wait until this technology is being used everywhere. We can try to become aware of current available systems and influence future implementation.

There are several reasons to be cautious. If data are written in a proprietary format that is not readily exported, we risk losing the effort made to enter the data. We must insist on open architecture or easy export of data. Unless upgrades are assured, software programs that are not compatible with mainframes or with the desktop PCs of tomorrow are dead-end investments. Both hardware and software require service, updates, and willingness of others in the hospital to buy in.

Available Programs

The American College of Emergency Physicians Section for Computers in Emergency Medicine has maintained a list of pertinent hardware and software. The listings in Tables 4.1 to 4.8 are adapted from their *Computer Software Directory*.

Physician Scheduling

Computers can transform the task of scheduling multiple physicians around rotating schedules. Many of these programs (Table 4.1) can keep track of personal preferences, vacation requests, and conflicting schedules. Some can keep track of and repair inequities.

Patient Charting

The medical chart is frequently difficult to read. The information is laboriously handwritten, frequently by a physician whose penmanship deteriorates from poor to unreadable as the shift progresses. Data can be spotty. Entering a record onto a computer has met with resistance from physicians whose typing skills are not up to the task. Real-time transcription can be costly.

Automated charting can produce a printed record on the fly. Some of these systems are voice-activated. In other cases, a touch-screen allows the production of a printed chart at the touch of a button. Some of the systems guide the dictation and demand input based on chief complaint (e.g., positive and negative risk factors for coronary vascular disease must be addressed for adult patients presenting with a chief complaint of chest pain). Others allow the physician to guide the input.

Whether using voice recognition, which is steadily increasing in sophistication and intelligence, touch-screen technology, or other modes of operation, these systems (Table 4.2) strive to offer alternatives to simply typing the record.

Diagnosis

Medical diagnosis by computer, though still in its infancy, is beginning to make its way into the clinical setting. The programs described in Table 4.3 may be of use to the emergency physician.

Pharmacy and Pharmacology

Current software (Table 4.4) excels. Computerized drug information allows for immediate access and simple cross-referencing of in-depth drug information. Patient complaints can easily be compared to extensive adverse reaction lists. Drug interactions can be prevented. Such software may also be placed on mainframe computers for access over hospital-wide information systems.

Patient Instructions

Discharge instructions are frequently cryptic and unintelligibly handwritten. The programs for generating printed discharge instructions listed in Table 4.5 allow uniformity in aftercare management. Table 4.6 lists software for QA and CQI applications.

Registration/Triage/Tracking

Patient tracking is replicated at several stages in the emergency department. In some institutions the triage nurse, Registration, the nursing station, and the discharge nurse all keep logs of their activities. Each enters the same patient data (name, registration number, time, and chief complaint). Despite this log keeping, departments also develop boards to keep track of the patient's location and stage of workup. Automated tracking (Table 4.7) eliminates this redundancy of effort.

Educational

Besides facilitating home study, computer-assisted instruction (CAI) allows for immediate training when unfamiliar problems or diagnoses are encountered. Programs loaded onto the computer do not "disappear" from a shelf. Furthermore, extensive libraries may be kept in much a smaller working area. Table 4.8 gives examples.

TABLE 4.1. Systems for automated physician scheduling

Name	Company	Description	Hardware	Cost
DOCS for Windows. (Dr on Call Schedule) Staff scheduling for call and daily assignments	Acme Express, Inc. 3311 Perkins Avenue Cleveland, OH 44144 216-391-7400 FAX: 216-391-0707 Don Scipione dscipione@acmex.com www.acmex.com	Generates and optimizes work schedules. Remembers past inequities and compensates in future assignments. Expertise groups. Teams. Same day assignments. Circadial profiles. Default on/off requests.	IBM PC 486+ Windows 3.11 or Windows 95 Microsoft Excel	$1500
EPSKED, Version 3.0 Physician scheduling	ByteBloc Medical Software 3102 Lilly Avenue Long Beach, CA 90808 562-596-5915 FAX 562-430-9400 Mark Boettger, MD, FACEP bytebloc@deltanet.com http://www.wp.com/bytebloc	Calendar display. Automates scheduling of up to 12 shifts/day, 40 MDs. Calculates summaries, does cycled scheduling, more. Free functional demo. Top rated in ACEP Section of Computers in Emergency Medicine 1992–1993 Software Review.	PC-type 500K free convention memory, 1 HD disk d DOS 3.1 or better; Mac w SoftPC or Soft Windows	$635
On Schedule Physician scheduling	R-Soft 217 Jefferson Road, Box E St Louis, MO 63119 314-968-8522 William Reinus, MD	Allows flexible scheduling of rotating personel in any desired time format. Tracks time scheduled. Allows workarounds of vacations, meetings, etc.		$160
Scheduleez 3D Physician scheduling	EMPCO P.O. Box 877 Bloomington, IL 61701 309-825-3672 Scott Januzik, MD, FACEP	An automated scheduler. Three-dimensional scheduler can handle up to 50 MDs in 4 locations, 10 shifts per location, up to 1 year at a time. Cumulative calculators, mouse-driven, block copy, more	PC-Compatible DOS 2.1 or later	$499
TeleMed ED Patient Documentation Syst Daily staff on-call scheduling	RLIS, Inc. 15600 San Pedro, Suite 203 San Antonio, Texas 78232 800-496-7547 Jerry Gerson, VP Marketing Per site evaluation 73500.1056@compuserv.com	The TeleMed System provides staff daily on call assignments, specialty specific, fully integrated with the TeleMed Patient Tracking and Documentation System (Patents pending) (See Multi-Module/ Integrated Systems) Multiterminal/Multiuser	Any Windows NT compatible hardware, NT Server, Windows NT	On request

TABLE 4.1. *Continued*

Name	Company	Description	Hardware	Cost
The Employee Schedule, Version 3 Physician scheduling	Practical Applications P.O. Box 115 North Washington, PA 16048 412-894-2044 Orrin Stitt	Enables use of computer to help prepare schedules, cuts time by 50–75%. Does not automatically schedule, but does allow copying of repeat schedules, prints individual, daily, weekly and biweekly schedules. Also prints assignment reports.	PC-Compatible w 512K, printer DOS 3.0 or better	$169
Who Works When Schedule generation	Newport Systems 636 120th Avenue, NE Bellevue, WA 98005 800-782-1233 FAX 206-455-4895 Karen Gray	Schedules employees to preset shifts in shift-oriented environments. Choose from job-code, station, and team parameters to schedule up to 200 employees. Schedule 1–6 weeks at a time. Can do automatic schedule rotations, patterns.	PC-Compat; 640K; HD; printer MS-DOS 3.0 or better	$395

TABLE 4.2. Systems for automated patient charting

Name	Company	Description	Hardware	Cost
ED Chartpad Portable patient charting using "touch screen" technology	Compass Systems Corporation 2714 Union Avenue, Ext D., Suite 305 Memphis, TN 38112 901-458-5732 FAX 901-458-0403 Errol Dunn/Glen Cummins	Touch or write to create comprehensive patient charts at bedside. No keyboard or mouse. Portable touch screen technology. 22 chief complaint templates, body illustrations, CPT/ICD coding, discharge instructions, Prescriptions statistical PC database.	386 IBM compatible PC and laser printer/486 IBM compatible Turnkey	$15,000– $35,000
EMStation Pen/Voice-generated patient charting, including Prescription	Datamedic Clinical Systems 20 Oser Avenue Hauppauge, NY 11788 800-446-4021 David Fetterolf URL www.datamedic.com	Voice, pen-tablet, mouse, and/or keyboard chart generation via Windows software. No need for writing or traditional transcription. User-modifiable menu-driven charting. Text displayed as you speak. ICD-9/CPT codes automatically generated. Internal FAX	Hardware is included. Software is included.	$38,000 single user

(Continued)

TABLE 4.2. *Continued*

Name	Company	Description	Hardware	Cost
Field Based Run Reporting Software Field based EMS run records	UCS, Inc. 2005 West Cypress Creek Road, Suite 1 Fort Lauderdale, FL 33309 305-771-8116 FAX: 305-771-8601 Tom Mersch tomm@ucsworks.com www.ucsworks.com E-mail	Designed to meet stringent EMS requirements for fast and accurate collection of data. UCS's "Fireman Friendly" user interface makes navigation between screens and entry of data quick to train and easy to use.	Laptop-or Pen-based 485 75 mhz and above Windows 3.1/95 NT Host	on request
Kurzweil Voice EM Voice-generated patient charting	Kurzweil Applied Intelligence 411 Waverly Oakes Road Waltham, MA 02154-9990 617-893-5151 FAX 617-893-6525 Roxane Brocato	50,000-work voice recognition report generator for producing ED charts quickly without handwriting or transcription. Prompts for RBRVS detailed histories. ICD-9, CPT-4 codes generated. Easy-to-use editor. QA and risk management software available.	486 with 32 MB RAM DOS 3.3 or higher	~$42,900
TeleMed ED Patient Documentation System Physician/Nurse charting system	RLIS, Inc. 15600 San Pedro, Suite 203 San Antonio, Texas 78232 800-496-7547 Jerry Gerson, VP Marketing 73500.1056@compuserv.com	Provides intuitive, comprehensive entry of all facets of the ED chart. Employing a multitude of information entry methods all optimized for speed and accuracy, TeleMed automatically creates complete records in plain English text compliant with HCFA.	Any Windows NT compatible hardware, NT Server, Windows NT	Per site evaluation

TABLE 4.3. Some software to aid in diagnosis

Name	Company	Description	Hardware	Cost
TeleMed ED Patient Documentation System Differential diagnoses from patient complaints	RLIS, Inc. 15600 San Pedro, Suite 203 San Antonio, Texas 78232 800-496-7547 Jerry Gerson, VP Marketing 73500.1056@compuserv.com	Provides structured differential diagnosis based on patient complaints, all diagnoses being age and sex specific, with the working differential diagnosis tailored to the specific patient. Multiple diagnoses are allowed. (Patents pending)	Any Windows NT compatible hardware, NT Server, Windows NT	Per site evaluation

TABLE 4.4. Pharmacy and pharmacology software

Name	Company	Description	Hardware	Cost
Emergi-Dos 3.0	L.A. Medsig 8021 Barocco Drive Harahan, LA 70123 504-738-1044 FAX: 504-738-7080 Charles Sea, MD	14 programs for calculating and physician/patient teaching. 14 compiled programs designed to assist the ED physician in treating a variety of conditions and in doing calculations, deriving drug dosages, and teaching both the physician and his patients.	IBM PC DOS	Shareware
I.V. CALC Intravenous drug calculator	CritiSoft Medical Software, Inc P.O. Box 6238 Newport News, VA 23606-6238 757-989-5309 FAX 757-989-5309 James A. Fish, Jr, MD, FACEP	Quickly/easily creates patient specific IV infusion drip charts. Legible, well-documented IV drip charts in seconds! No training time. Fully supports 20 drugs—from aminophyllin to vasopressin. Universal mode that will create drip charts for ANY drug!	IBM PC, XT, AT, PS/2, or compatible with 384K RA DOS 2.1 or later	$295
Drug Guide 1.0 Drug interactions and side effects	Patient Medical Records, Inc 901 Tahoka Road Brownfield, TX 79316-3899 800-285-7627 Kelly Terry, Marketing Manager pmrincorp@aol.com pmrinc.com	Indexes 2,500 drugs with interactions and side effects. 550 diseases that affect therapy can be considered. Includes interactions and side effects for prescription and OTC drugs as well as many foods. Most recent update, April, 1997	IBM PC; 512K RAM, HD	$49.95 Update $25.00
DRUG-REAX™ Interactive system on drug interections	Micromedex, Inc. 6200 South Syracuse Way, Suite 300 Englewood, CO 80111-4740 303-486-6400 800-525-9083 Nancy Sayre info@mdx.com	Allows clinician to check interacting drug ingredients, effects, and clinical significance. Checks drug–drug, drug–food, drug–disease, drug–ethanol, and drug–laboratory assay interactions, plus previous allergic reactions.	AT-Compatible w 640K; color; CD-ROM drive DOS 3.3 or better	

(Continued)

TABLE **4.4.** *Continued*

Name	Company	Description	Hardware	Cost
DRUGDEX® General drug information system	Micromedex, Inc. 6200 South Syracuse Way, Suite 300 Englewood, CO 80111-4740 303-486-6400 800-525-9083 Nancy Sayre info@mdx.com	Unbiased drug information system. Includes over 1300 drug eval monographs and 5800 drug consults. Prescription, OTC, and investigational drugs included. Indexed by brand and generic name as well as disease state.	AT-Compatible w 640K; color; CD-ROM drive DOS 3.3 or better	
Electronic Drug Reference General drug information and patient advice	Clinical Reference Systems Ltd. 7100 Belleview Avenue, Suite 208 Greenwood Village, CO 80111 800-237-8401 FAX 303-220-1685 Sales Department crs-info@cliniref.com	Synthesis of drug data from six major references. Allows search of indications, dosages, adverse effects, etc., for over 5000 drugs. Includes advice in lay language which can be printed for handout.	PC-compatible; 640K RAM; 5.2 MB HD DOS 3.0 or better	$495
IDENTIDEX® Pill identification system	Micromedex, Inc. 6200 South Syracuse Way, Suite 300 Englewood, CO 80111-4740 303-486-6400 800-525-9083 Nancy Sayre info@mdx.com	Tablet and capsule identification system. Uses manufacturers' imprint code as well as color, shape, etc. Both prescription and OTC drugs. Also includes street drugs and slang names.	AT-Compat w 640K; color; CD-ROM drive DOS 3.3 or better	
IV Incompatibility Module (IVIM) Intravenous drug compatibilities	First Data Bank 1111 Bayhill Drive, Suite 350 San Bruno, CA 94066 800-633-3453 Marketing Department	Checks IV drug-to-IV drug and IV drug-to-IV solution compatibilities. Updated quarterly.	PC-Compatible; about 4MB HD DOS 2.0 or better	$480/year
Med Letter Drug Interactions Program Drug interactions	Medical Letter 1000 Main Street New Rochelle, NY 10801 914-235-0500 Ms. Pamela J. Scagnelli, Customer Service	This program allows input of multiple medications and flags potential interactions.	PC Compatible, Macintosh (See Vendor for specific DOS, Windows, Mac Version 6.0.5 or later)	

TABLE **4.4.** *Continued*

Name	Company	Description	Hardware	Cost
Medicom Micro PC Drug interactions	Professional Drug Systems, Inc. 530 Maryville Center Drive, Suite 250 St. Louis, MO 63141 800-366-4737	Identifies potential interactions between two or more medications along with a "significance code" ranging from 1 to 9.	IBM PC with 20MB HD	$695 + $40/month or $75/ quarter
PDR Electronic Library Computer version of entire PDR	Medical Economics 5 Paragon Drive Montvale, NJ 07645 800-232-7379 PDR Electronics Customer Service	The complete library of PDR products on CD-Rom. Also available with other modules such as Merck Manual $99.95, Stedman's Medical Dictionary $79.95, Stedman's Spell Check $99.95, Griffith's 5 Minute Clinical Consult $59.95, and PDR Drug ID $39.95.	PC-Compatible DOS 3.0 or better or Windows 3.1 or better	$595 ($535 for renewals)
PDR's Drug Interactions, Side Effects and Interactions PDR's drug interactions and side effects system	Medical Economics 5 Paragon Drive Montvale, NJ 07645 800-232-7379 PDR Electronics Customer Service	Allows user to check multidrug regimens for interactions or to check a particular drug for indications, side effects, or interactions with any other drug(s). Stores drug regimens for individual patients that can be retrieved, updated, and rechecked.	PC-Compatible DOS 3.0 or better	$235 ($155 for updates)
Pharmaceuticals 3.0 DOS, MAC, or palmtop drug reference	ComputerBooks P.O. Box 9167 Newport Beach, CA 92658 800-848-2023	Covers the 250 top selling pharmaceutical agents. Includes trade and generic names, FDA prescribing information with warnings, dosage, route of administration, FDA approved and nonapproved indications, contraindications, and adverse reactions.	PC, MAC, or HP palmtop DOS 3.0 or better; DOS emulator for use on MAC	$199

(Continued)

TABLE **4.4.** *Continued*

Name	Company	Description	Hardware	Cost
RxTriage Drug interactions with patient advise	First Data Bank 1111 Bayhill Drive, Suite 350 San Bruno, CA 94066 800-633-3453 Marketing Department	Performs drug interaction assessment with estimation of relative risk. Also does drug-to-food interactions, prints ASHP patient instruction leaflets, and checks for duplicate therapies. Updated quarterly.	IBM PC with 2.5 MB HD	$480/year
SOAP Drug Interaction Program Drug interactions and side effects	Patient Medical Records, Inc. 901 Tahoka Road Brownfield, TX 79316-3899 800-285-7627 Kelly Terry, Marketing Manager pmrincorp@aol.com	Drug interaction software that includes a prescription writer. Will list all side effects of an individual drug color coded for level of frequency. Does not require a hard drive. Most recent update, April, 1997.	IBM PC	$199.50 + $90/update
TeleMed ED Patient Documentation System evaluation Prescriptions and medication orders	RLIS, Inc. 15600 San Pedro, Suite 203 San Antonio, Texas 78232 800-496-7547 Jerry Gerson, VP Marketing 73500.1056@compuserv.com	Provides exceptionally fast generation of prescriptions or medication orders in the ED. Physician-specific customization is included. Selection of drugs for inclusion comes from a 28,000 drug database. Formulary specific filters are included.	Any Windows NT compatible hardware, NT Server, Windows NT	Per site evaluation

TABLE 4.5. Automated patient instruction systems

Name	Company	Description	Hardware	Cost
Adult Health Advisor Patient instructions	Clinical Reference Systems Ltd. 7100 Belleview Avenue, Suite 208 Greenwood Village, CO 80111 800-237-8401 FAX 303-220-1685 Sales Department crs-info@cliniref.com	Provides patient advice on over 500 medical/surgical topics. Can be used to print user-modifiable handouts.	PC-Compatible; 640K RAM; 3 MB HD DOS 3.0 or better	$395
Behavioral Health Advisor Patient Instructions	Clinical Reference Systems, Ltd. 7100 Belleview Avenue, Suite 208 Greenwood Village, CO 80111 800-237-8401 FAX 303-220-1685 Sales Department crs-info@cliniref.com	Patient advice handouts on common adult and pediatric behavioral and mental health topics. Can be modified by user.	PC-Compatible; 640K RAM; 1.5 MB HD DOS 3.0 or better	$395
Care Notes™ Patient instructions	Micromedex, Inc. 6200 South Syracuse Way, Suite 300 Englewood, CO 80111-4740 303-486-6400 800-525-9083 Nancy Sayre info@mdx.com www.micromedex.com	Provides patient discharge instructions. Customized. Includes facility name, treating MD, date, patient name, explanation of injury/illness, guidelines for self-care, further followup. Available in English/Spanish	AT-Compatible w 640K; color; CD-ROM drive	
CEPIS— After Care System Patient instructions, scripts, follow-up, statistics	MedAmerica Information Services 588 Blossom Hill Road San Jose, CA 95123 408-988-0891 FAX 408-365-8579 Benjamin Young	Generates detailed patient discharge instructions (English or other languages) with detachable prescriptions. Tracks patient followup, prints summary and statistical reports. Additional module available which allows additional query functions.	PC 486/ Pentium, 16 MB Ram, 200 MB HD Microsoft Windows (LAN optional) NT	$895

(Continued)

TABLE 4.5. *Continued*

Name	Company	Description	Hardware	Cost
Checkout™ **LOGICARE** **Level I** **System** Patient instructions, releases, and built-in Q.A. Q.A.	LOGICARE Corporation P.O. Box 224 Eau Claire, WI 54702-0224 800-848-0099 Judy Adams, Sales Analyst solver@logicare.com E-mail: WWW url:	Installed in over 300 Emergency Departments, CHECKOUT patient instructions have 900 adult and pediatric topics. Also includes prescriptions, miscellaneous forms, and optional English/Spanish side-by-side instructions. Easily customized; expandable.	IBM Compatible p-133 or better Windows 95/NT	$5450 (1st copy), $2400 (add-on)
EDDS-ED **Discharge** **System** Patient discharge instructions	CYBIS Medical Systems, Inc. 1601 114th Avenue SE, Suite 103 Bellevue, WA 98004 800-336-1042 FAX: 206-453-4502 Lisa Lester, Product Manager 76011.142@compuserve.com	Discharge instructions, practice management, and reporting. EDDS contains 1600 diagnoses that include ICD-9 codes and over 200 medications. Text is written by board-certified emergency physicians, and reviewed for 6th grade or lower reading level.	IBM Compatible PC 40MB HD Network option available DOS, Windows, Windows 95, OS/2 versions available	$3795
Emer Pt **Instruction** **Compiler** Patient instructions	Epic Software Systems Inc 7498 Upper Applegate Road Jacksonville, OR 97530 541-770-1726 FAX 541-899-8721 Earl Showerman, MD, FACEP epic@mind.net	Over 300 sites installed, more than 10 years of development and experience. Prescription writer and network application planned for future releases.	PC 386 or better; 640K RAM; 20MB HD for version Windows 95 for version 5.0	$1000 discounts available
EMpro Instructions, scripts, excuses, referrals, billing, and QA	E.I.S., Inc. P.O. Box 13703 RTP, NC 27709 800-605-6241 919-544-3580	Registration information downloaded from mainframe. Light pen used to pick Dx's, Rx's, excuses, and charges. Creates laser printed set of aftercare instructions, scripts, work and school excuses, physician referrals, and ICD-9/CPT charges. Automated billing and CQI.	486, 8 MB RAM, 200MBHD, 14.4 modem, laser printer DOS 6.2, Close Up	$15,500

TABLE 4.5. *Continued*

Name	Company	Description	Hardware	Cost
Exit-Writer! Patient instructions	Parker Hill Associates 987 Airway Court, Suite 20 Santa Rosa, CA 95403 800-598-7258 FAX 707-525-1339 David Campell, MD, FACEP parker@wco.com www.exit-writer.com	Over 500 instruction topics: illnesses and injuries, medications, diets and appliances, consent forms, school and work releases. Referral MD and phrase list. Spanish translations. Built-in editor. Full Windows support. Free product updates and phone support.	MS-DOS or Windows 3.1/ Workgroups/ 95/NT	$3495
Homecare Personalized homecare instruction sheets and log function	EM Alternatives, Inc. P.O. Box 152 Mequon, WI 53092 800-909-3624 Cynthia McGirr	Allows a nurse to provide printed copy of personalized instructions using standard protocol that has been reviewed by medical experts. Updated annually. Log function allows to sort by patient name, date of visit, doctor, nurse, medications, or protocol used.	IBM-Compatible, 3.5″ diskette 1.5 mb of storage, DOS	$295
HomeEasy-Discharge Instruction Package Discharge Instructions, Rx's, Log	Wellsoft Corporation 605 Franklin Boulevard, Suite 5 Somerset, NJ 08873 800-597-9909 Denise Helfand, Marketing Director	2000 illnesses, drugs, surgeries, tests and diagnostic procedure sheets—includes Spanish sheets, drug/drug and drug/ food interactions, Rx's and work/ school releases. Offered separately or as part of Integrated Package. Includes standard JCAHO log.	PC-Compatible; 486/33 4meg RAM, 270mb HD or bet Networkable, Turn-key available. Dos/Windows Version	$5000 1st Unit, $3500 Add-On
Medication Advisor Specific medication advice for patients	Clinical Reference Systems, Ltd. 7100 Belleview Avenue, Suite 208 Greenwood Village, CO 80111 800-237-8401 FAX 303-220-1685 Sales Department crs-info@cliniref.com	Generates two-page patient advice sheets for over 5000 drugs, both prescription and OTC. Can be personalized for each physician and patient.	PC-Compatible; 640K RAM; 1.9 MB HD DOS 3.0 or better	$395

(Continued)

TABLE **4.5.** *Continued*

Name	Company	Description	Hardware	Cost
PAIGE Patient Instruction Generator Discharge instruction editor and printer. Prints scripts.	Mad Scientist Software 115 E. 200 North Alpine, UT 84004 800-250-2988 FAX: 801-763-9925 Dominic Bria madsci19@idt.net www.madsci.com	Simple aftercare instruction program. Pick diagnosis, drug, treatment, and followup instructions from database. Packaged 1200 instructions are easily edited. Links treatment plans. Prints prescriptions and standard forms. Spanish instructions available.	PC-Compatible; printer DOS, Windows	$289.95 + $150 for Spanish
Pediatric Advisor Pediatric patient instructions	Clinical Reference Systems Ltd. 7100 Belleview Avenue, Suite 208 Greenwood Village, CO 80111 800-237-8401 FAX 303-220-1685 Sales Department crs-info@cliniref.com	Provides advice to parents on over 800 infant, child, and adolescent problems, including clinical issues, divorce, newborn care, etc. Can be edited. Generates handouts on these topics with many illustrations. Available with Spanish translations.	PC-Compatible; 640K RAM; 2.7 MB HD DOS 3.0 or better	$395 ($595 Spanish/ English Version)
ScriptSure Patient instructions and prescription writer for ambulatory care	DAW Systems 47 Sweet Road Ballston Lake, NY 12019 800-348-9899	Designed for outpatient care settings. Includes prescription writing, treatment instructions, medication summaries, memo writing for patient instructions, laboratory and x-ray orders, medication information for physicians, school/ work release forms, and autodialing.	PC 386; 2MB RAM; 5MB HD + 1MB per 500 patient MS-DOS	$3995

TABLE **4.5.** *Continued*

Name	Company	Description	Hardware	Cost
Senior Health Advisor Patient instructions	Clinical Reference Systems, Ltd. 7100 E. Belleview Avenue, Suite 208 Greenwood Village, CO 80111 800-237-8401 FAX 303-220-1685 Sales Department crs-info@cliniref.com	Provides patient advice on over 275 topics covering a broad range of geriatric health topics, including biomedical, psychological, and social issues encounted in older healthcare.	PC-Compatible; 640K RAM; 2MB HD DOS 3.0 or better	$395
TeleMed ED Patient Documenta-tion System Patient instructions	PLIS, Inc. 15600 San Pedro, Suite 203 San Antonio, Texas 78232 800-496-7547 Jerry Gerson, VP Marketing 73500.1056@compuserv.com	Automatically creates custom set of patient instructions based on the diagnoses, treatment rendered, patient referral, prescriptions given. Instructions automatically list treating physician, date/time, facility, w/patient signature page. (Patents pending)	Any Windows NT compatible hardware, NT Server, Windows NT	Per site evaluation
Women's Health Advisor Patient instructions	Clinical Reference Systems Ltd. 7100 Belleview Avenue, Suite 208 Greenwood Village, CO 80111 800-237-8401 FAX 303-220-1685 Sales Department crs-info@cliniref.com	Provides patient advice on over 500 medical/surgical topics. Can be used to print user-modifiable handouts.	PC-Compatible; 640K RAM; 3.0 MB HD DOS 3.0 or better	$395

TABLE 4.6. Automated systems for QA and CQI

Name	Company	Description	Hardware	Cost
Chart Review Quality assurance software	Kurzweil Applied Intelligence 411 Waverley Oaks Road Waltham, MA 02154 617-893-5151 FAX 617-893-6525 Roxane Brocato	A QA software package to assist in analyzing VoiceEM charts for documentation. Design your own search criteria or use predefined templates. Print reports with reviewer's comments. ICD-9 analysis. Fast and easy to use.	IBM-Compatible DOS	$2500
Collector Trauma, coding, log, QA, research	Tri-Analytics, Inc 23 Ellendale Street, Suite A Bel Air, MD 21014 410-879-6767 ext 105 Douglas J. O'Bryon, MBA www.trianalytics.com	Provides tools to accumulate patient data and generate QA and research reports and queries. Trauma registry accomodates ACS, CDC, and JCAHO audit filters. TRICODE coding software included.	PC-Compatible; 640K; HD DOS 5.0 or better, Windows 3.1/95/NT	$5000 plus $1500/ year lease
E Qual QA Modules for specific clinical topics	ED Logic 2280 Elmhill Road Pittsburgh, PA 15221 412-731-0467	A series of approximately 20 modules, each of which allows ED QA for a clinical topic. Examples are AMA, Chest Pain, Deaths within 48 hours. Also includes several EMS topics.	PC-Compatible w 512K, HD, Color, Printer DOS 2.1 or better	$90 per module
EMERGE™ Emergency Patient Care Resource Management	Medicus Systems Corporation One Rotary Center, Suite 1111 Evanston, IL 60201 847-570-7500; 888-MEDICUS Elena Arrigo, Marketing Manager info@ccmail.medicus.com www.medicus.com	ED staffing system designed for workload measurement, workload trending, productivity reporting, and budget development.	IBM-Compatible PC	Please see vendor
LOGICARE Level II System System for emergency data tracking	LOGICARE Corporation P.O. Box 224 Eau Claire, WI 54702-0224 800-848-0099 Judy Adams, Sales Analyst solver@logicare.com	Customized installations automate the ED log and become the core of ED data tracking. Includes discharge instructions, report writer, statistics, quality assurance capabilities, interface to hospital computer. Expandable to LOGICARE Level III.	IBM-Compatible 486 or better DOS 5 or higher; Windows 3.1 or higher	$28,200–$58,200

TABLE 4.6. *Continued*

Name	Company	Description	Hardware	Cost
LOGICARE Level III System Emergency Patient Tracking	LOGICARE Corporation P.O. Box 224 Eau Claire, WI 54702-0224 800-848-0099 Judy Adams, Sales Analyst solver@logicare.com	Customized installations- Level II plus expanded electronic log, detailed patient flow and customized tracking boards, real-time and retrospective report generation, QA, registration, order entry and results reporting interfaces, MD dictation storage and retrieval.	IBM-Compatible 486 or better DOS 5 or higher; Windows 3.1 or higher	$95,000–$132,000
TeleMed ED Patient Documentation System QA and CQI	RLIS, Inc. 15600 San Pedro, Suite 203 San Antonio, Texas 78232 800-496-7547 Jerry Gerson, VP Marketing 73500.1056@compuserv.com	Creates an unlimited array of reports dealing with high-risk diagnoses, treatment time statistics, disease surveillance statistics, automatic trauma registry, concurrent checking for complete data collection, automatic date/time stamping of events.	Any Windows NT compatible hardware, NT Server, Windows NT	Per site evaluation
Trauma Registry Coding Guide Trauma registry	Centers for Disease Control Biometrics Branch Atlanta, GA 30333	This is a combination software package and guidebook from the CDC. It is the result of a large 1988 conference, and is designed to encourage unifrom trauma registries nationwide. Send five 5 1/4 360K blank disks with SASE.		Free
Tri-Code Trauma coding and QA	Tri-Analytics 23 Ellendale St, Suite A Bel Air, MD 21014 410-879-6767 ext 105 Douglas J. O'Bryon, MBA	Designed for medical records and trauma care providers. Allows consistent coding of text descriptions of injury into ICD-9-CM and AIS85 or AIS90. Useful for trauma systems studies, research, and QA.	PC-Compatible; 640K; HD DOS 5.0 or better	$975/year lease

TABLE 4.7. Automated systems for registration, tracking, and triage

Name	Company	Description	Hardware	Cost
CATS (Computer Assisted Triage System) Algorithm-directed computerized triage and screening with paging option	IPI Health Systems 5332 South Memorial, #200 Tulsa, OK 74145 USA 918-624-9284 FAX: 918-492-6237 Paul D. Bradford, Technical Director	Allows doctors, nurses, medical technicians, RNs, or physian assistants to effectively screen, triage, and identify patients requiring immediate care from those who can be treated less urgently. Available in all foreign languages supported by Microsoft.	IBM PC and laptop, compatibles, laptops, and servers DOS 3.3–6.2. Windows compatible, ProComm compatible	$1500 initial setup/ $600 annual
LOGICARE Level II System System for emergency data tracking	LOGICARE Corporation P.O. Box 224 Eau Claire, WI 54702-0224 800-848-0099 Judy Adams, Sales Analyst solver@logicare.com	Customized installations automate the ED log and become the core of ED data tracking. Includes discharge instructions, report writer, statistics, quality assurance capabilities, interface to hospital computer. Expandable to LOGICARE Level III.	IBM-Compatible 486 or better DOS 5 or higher; Windows 3.1 or higher	$28,200–$58,200
LOGICARE Level III System Emergency Patient Tracking	LOGICARE Corporation P.O. Box 224 Eau Claire, WI 54702-0224 800-848-0099 Judy Adams, Sales Analyst solver@logicare.com	Customized installations—Level II plus expanded electronic log, detailed patient flow and customized tracking boards, real-time and retrospective report generation, QA, registration, order entry and results reporting interfaces, MD dictation storage and retrieval.	IBM-Compatible 486 or better DOS 5 or higher; Windows 3.1 or higher	$95,000–$132,000
MDE EDCoder™ Coding, Transcription, Quality Assurance and Information Management	MDE, Inc. 4 Foster Avenue, Suite A Gibbsboro, NJ 08026 609-784-4300 FAX 609-784-8412 Joanne L. Snow Jsnow@MDEonline.com	MDE provides coding, transcription, and CQI exclusively for ED records. Voice prompted system, with real-time coding feedback on every chart, helps physicians meet documentation requirements and contributes to increase revenues 23%–40%		Varies—Coding priced per chart

TABLE **4.7.** *Continued*

Name	Company	Description	Hardware	Cost
TeleMed ED Patient Documentation System Tracking	RLIS, Inc. 15600 San Pedro, Suite 203 San Antonio, Texas 78232 800-496-7547 Jerry Gerson, VP Marketing 73500.1056@compuserv.com	Tracks all patients in the ED. Multiple views of patient data including a unique ED layout view are provided. Laboratory, x-ray, order, and reevaluation status are constantly updated. A unique "pending orders" screen streamlines ED communication.	Any Windows NT compatible hardware, NT Server, Windows NT	Per site evaluation
TeleMed ED Patient Documentation System Triage	RLIS, Inc. 15600 San Pedro, Suite 203 San Antonio, Texas 78232 800-496-7547 Jerry Gerson, VP Marketing 73500.1056@compuserv.com	Leads ED personnel through triage and rapidly produces a superlative, accurate, useable, defendable triage assessment. Triage time is reduced and can be accomplished anywhere in the ED. Laboratory and x-ray ordering can be entered at triage. (Patent pending)	Any Windows NT compatible hardware, NT Server, Windows NT	Per site evaluation
TeleMed ED Patient Documentation System Daily Visit Log	RLIS, Inc. 15600 San Pedro, Suite 203 San Antonio, Texas 78232 800-496-7547 Jerry Gerson, VP Marketing 73500.1056@compuserv.com	Automatically generate complete ED registration and discharge logs meeting and exceeding all JCAHO requirements. Statistics are complied into reports covering any user-defined period. Payor mix reports and physician specific logs can be printed.	Any Windows NT compatible hardware, NT Server, Windows NT	Per site evaluation

TABLE **4.8.** Educational software

Name	Company	Description	Hardware	Cost
Abdominal Pain: Exercises in Clinical Problem Solving Abdominal Pain	Williams and Wilkins 351 West Camden Street Baltimore, MD 21201-2346 800-527-5597 Robert Mason custserv@wwilkins.com	The RxDx series. One of fifteen educational software packages, which involve interactive education by managing simulated patients.	IBM PC, 256K RAM, HD or 2 floppies DOS 2.0 or higher	$375
Adv Prob Cardiac Arrhythmias Cardiac arrhythmias	Williams and Wilkins 351 West Camden Street Baltimore, MD 21201-2346 800-527-5597 Robert Mason custserv@wwilkins.com	The RxDx series. One of fifteen educational software packages which involve interactive education by managing simulated patients.	IBM PC, 256K RAM, HD or 2 floppies DOS 2.0 or higher	$375
Anemia: Exercises in Clinical Problem Solving Anemia	Williams and Wilkins 351 West Camden Street Baltimore, MD 21201-2346 800-527-5597 Robert Mason custserv@wwilkins.com	The RxDx series. One of fifteen educational software packages which involve interactive education by managing simulated patients.	IBM PC, 256K RAM, HD or 2 floppies DOS 2.0 or higher	$375
Arrhythmias Tutorial Part I and II Cardiac arrhythmias	Williams and Wilkins 351 West Camden Street Baltimore, MD 21201-2346 800-527-5597 Robert Mason custserv@wwilkins.com	The RxDx series. One of fifteen educational software packages which involve interactive education by managing simulated patients.	IBM PC, 256K RAM, HD or 2 floppies DOS 2.0 or higher	$375
Arrhythmias: Case Studies in Management Cardiac arrhythmias	Williams and Wilkins 351 West Camden Street Baltimore, MD 21201-2346 800-527-5597 Robert Mason custserv@wwilkins.com	The RxDx series. One of fifteen educational software packages which involve interactive education by managing simulated patients.	IBM PC, 256K RAM, HD or 2 floppies DOS 2.0 or higher	$375
Arterial Blood Gases Arterial blood gases	Williams and Wilkins 351 West Camden Street Baltimore, MD 21201-2346 800-527-5597 Robert Mason custserv@wwilkins.com	The RxDx series. One of fifteen educational software packages which involve interactive education by managing simulated patients.	IBM PC, 256K RAM, HD or 2 floppies DOS 2.0 or higher	$375
Basic Life Support BLS	Williams and Wilkins 351 West Camden Street Baltimore, MD 21201-2346 800-527-5597 Robert Mason custserv@wwilkins.com	The RxDx series. One of fifteen educational software packages which involve interactive education by managing simulated patients.	IBM PC, 256K RAM, HD or 2 floppies DOS 2.0 or higher	$375
Bleeding Disorders: Exercises in Clinical Problem Solving Bleeding disorders	Williams and Wilkins 351 West Camden Street Baltimore, MD 21201-2346 800-527-5597 Robert Mason custserv@wwilkins.com	The RxDx series. One of fifteen educational software packages which involve interactive education by managing simulated patients.	IBM PC, 256K RAM, HD or 2 floppies DOS 2.0 or higher	$375

TABLE **4.8.** *Continued*

Name	Company	Description	Hardware	Cost
Blood Gases Arterial blood gases	Mad Scientist Software 115 East 200 North Alpine, UT 84004 800-250-2988 FAX: 801-763-9925 Dominic Bria madsci19@idt.net www.madsci.com	Interactive program teaches ABG interp and analysis, including acid-base balance, treatment, A-a gradients.	PC-Compatible DOS, Windows	$69.95
Cardiac Arrest!—ACLS Teaching ACLS	Mad Scientist Software 115 East 200 North Alpine, UT 84004 800-250-2988 FAX: 801-763-9925 Dominic Bria madsci19@idt.net www.madsci.com	User plays role of emergency physician and directs a resuscitation. Enter orders in regular English. On-screen monitor strips, ABG results, etc. Critiques performance. Includes unusual arrests (hypothermia, etc.) Multiple student capabilities.	PC-Compatible DOS, Windows	$89.95
Cardiac Emergency Simulator ACLS	Cardinal Health Systems 4600 West 77th St, Suite 150 Edina, MN 55435 800-328-0180 Don Aaser	Generates real-time cardiac emergencies. User learns ACLS according to AHA protocols. Accredited for CME.	PC-Compatible DOS 2.1 or better	$149
Chest Pain Simulator Chest pain workup and thrombolytic therapy simulator	Mad Scientist Software 115 East 200 North Alpine, UT 84004 800-250-2988 FAX: 801-763-9925 Dominic Bria madsci19@idt.net www.madsci.com	Simulates the stabilization and workup of chest pain patients; take history, examine, order tests, intervene. Computer looks for weaknesses in approach. Practice thrombolytic indications and contraindications. Multiple student capabilities.	PC-Compatible DOS, Windows	$99.95
Chest Pain: Exercises in Clinical Problem Solving Chest pain	Williams and Wilkins 351 West Camden Street Baltimore, MD 21201-2346 800-527-5597 Robert Mason custserv@wwilkins.com	The RxDx series. One of fifteen educational software packages which involve interactive education by managing simulated patients.	IBM PC, 256K RAM, HD or 2 floppies DOS 2.0 or higher	$375
Code Team! ACLS	Mad Scientist Software 115 East 200 North Alpine, UT 84004 800-250-2988 FAX: 801-763-9925 Dominic Bria madsci19@idt.net www.madsci.com	Three-part program: CardioQuiz is 10 self-teaching ACLS quizzes; EKG teaches rhythms; ACLS Protocols reviews AHA protocols and presents test cases for management. Multiple student capabilities. Latest AHA standards.	PC-Compatible DOS, Windows	$79.95

TABLE 4.8. *Continued*

Name	Company	Description	Hardware	Cost
CPR Training by Computer CPR	Williams and Wilkins 351 West Camden Street Baltimore, MD 21201-2346 800-527-5597 Robert Mason custserv@wwilkins.com	The RxDx series. One of fifteen educational software packages which involve interactive education by managing simulated patients.	IBM PC, 256K RAM, HD or 2 floppies DOS 2.0 or higher	$375
Critical Care Medicine Acute MI Acute MI	Williams and Wilkins 351 West Camden Street Baltimore, MD 21201-2346 800-527-5597 Robert Mason custserv@wwilkins.com	The RxDx series. One of fifteen educational software packages which involve interactive education by managing simulated patients.	IBM PC, 256K RAM, HD or 2 floppies DOS 2.0 or higher	$375
Hypertension Management 2.0 Hypertension	Williams and Wilkins 351 West Camden Street Baltimore, MD 21201-2346 800-527-5597 Robert Mason custserv@wwilkins.com	The RxDx series. One of fifteen educational software packages which involve interactive education by managing simulated patients.	IBM PC, 256K RAM, HD or 2 floppies DOS 2.0 or higher	$375
Hypertensive Emergencies Hypertension	Williams and Wilkins 351 West Camden Street Baltimore, MD 21201-2346 800-527-5597 Robert Mason custserv@wwilkins.com	The RxDx series. One of fifteen educational software packages which involve interactive education by managing simulated patients.	IBM PC, 256K RAM, HD or 2 floppies DOS 2.0 or higher	$375
MD-Challenger V3.0 for Acute Care and Emergency Medicine Comprehensive clinical reference and training software	Challenger Corporation 5530 Summer Avenue Memphis, TN 38134 800-676-0822 FAX 901-385-8380 Dan Jones, MD, FACEP	Combines comprehensive interactive education with clinical reference. Approximately 4000 questions are integrated with 500 high resolution computed based images into 26 clinical chapters. The detailed index eases rapid search of the knowledge base.	PC: 4MB RAM,25 MB HD space; MAC: 4MB RAM, PC: Windows 3.1 or better; MAC: System 6.02 or b	$395 to 995 (includes CME)
MicroEKG 12-lead EKG interpretation	Mad Scientist Software 115 East 200 North Alpine, UT 84004 800-250-2988 FAX: 801-763-8925 Dominic Bria madsci19@idt.net www.madsci.com	Complete 12-lead EKG trainer: lead placement, wave forms, intervals, rhythms and arrythmias, chamber enlargement, conduction blockage, infarcts, ischemia. Multiple student capabilities.	PC-Compatible DOS, Windows	$89.95
Stupor and Coma: Exercises in Clinical Problem Solving Stupor and coma	Williams and Wilkins 351 West Camden Street Baltimore, MD 21201-2346 800-527-5597 Robert Mason custserv@wwilkins.com	The RxDx series. One of fifteen educational software packages which involve interactive education by managing simulated patients.	IBM PC, 256K RAM, HD or 2 floppies DOS 2.0 or higher	$375

TABLE **4.8.** *Continued*

Name	Company	Description	Hardware	Cost
Trauma One! Multiple trauma	Mad Scientist Software 115 East 200 North Alpine, UT 84004 800-250-2988 FAX: 801-763-9925 Dominic Bria madsci19@idt.net www.madsci.com	User manages multiple trauma patients, collecting historical and physical exam data, ordering tests and interventions. Teaches ABCs, priorities, completeness. Helpful preparation for oral boards. Extra patient disks available. Multiple student capabilities.	PC-Compatible DOS, Windows	$109.95–$139.95 Deluxe

5
Informatics in Emergency Radiology

Michael E. Flisak

Since Roentgen's first use of the x-ray almost 100 years ago, the radiographic film has been a key element used to communicate information about normal and pathologic anatomy and pathologic states in medicine. Its role in the emergency department (ED) has been extensive; the majority of traumatized patients undergo one or more imaging studies. We have traditionally relied on the x-ray film to capture, store, and transfer information between and among the radiology technologists, the radiologists, the managing emergency department physician, and paramedical personnel. To date, even primarily digital modalities such as computerized tomography (CT) and ultrasound (US) have relied on x-ray film as their short- and long-term storage and communication medium. Despite the benefits that have accrued over the years because of the use of x-ray films in medicine, there remain several inherent weaknesses in the use of this medium for imaging. These include its limited ability to capture x-ray photons, its physical characteristics and processing requirements, and its uniqueness as a physical entity. Changes in any one of these areas could significantly influence the use of x-rays and x-ray film in the hospital emergency department.

As a primary capturer of x-ray photons, x-ray film is an extremely inefficient medium. The silver halide grains present in the photographic emulsion utilize only a fraction of the x-ray energy that strikes them. This physical limitation has required the development of light-emitting and -intensifying film–screen systems that enhance efficiency, maintain resolution, decrease exposure time (and thus image unsharpness), and decrease radiation exposure to the patient. Film–screen systems are contained in the radiographic cassettes so familiar wherever radiographs are obtained.

Once x-ray absorption information has been stored in the silver halide granules on the film, processing is required to make this information visible in the form of a radiographic image. While much progress has been made over the years, film processing still requires relatively expensive equipment, uses toxic chemicals that must be disposed of, and takes a relatively long time to accomplish. Even high speed laser imagers utilize x-ray film and are subject to the same drawbacks.

If one could completely eliminate the foregoing problems, other limitations would remain, including long- and short-term storage requirements and transportation requirements. One of the greatest limitations of x-ray film is its uniqueness. Unless copies are made, only one instance of a given radiographic image exists in reality. It cannot be in different physical locations simultaneously, and it cannot be viewed simultaneously by different physicians in different physical locations.

The advent of digital imaging formats, which utilize high speed computers, point-to-point data transfer, and medium resolution television displays in the form of CT and US, sparked interest in the development of electronic imaging and electronic image transfer. Conceptually, a digitally stored image that can be transmitted over an electronic network eliminates many of the drawbacks inherent in x-ray film. Such a system has existed conceptually for 15 years and was originally termed a picture-archiving and communications system (PACS). Since data and images from CT, US, and magnetic resonance imaging (MRI) originate in digital format, adaptation of these modalities to a PACS environment would seem to be a small step. A larger hurdle might exist in the conversion of the analog information contained on "film" to a digital format or the development of technology to allow direct digital capture of an x-ray image, eliminating film altogether.

If and when a completely electronic digital imaging system comes to exist (encompassing all imaging modalities), it will have a major impact on patient throughput, diagnosis, and management in an ED setting, where time is often a critical factor. This chapter details the development of PACS systems over the past 10 to 15 years and discusses the future of radiology informatics in a filmless PACS environment.

Communication Protocols

The development of a filmless environment is a long and arduous process that has not yet been completed. While several proprietary systems are now in operation, it is extremely unusual today for one manufacturer to provide all the x-ray equipment used in an institution. Even if the necessary hardware, network technology, high resolution display monitors, and direct digital acquisition systems were developed at present, they could not be combined into a functional system from multiple vendors. For PACS systems to be successful, they must be able to acquire image data from a variety of imaging devices provided by a variety of manufacturers and subsequently to integrate this information into a cohesive PACS database.

Beginning in 1983, the American College of Radiology (ACR) in conjunction with the National Electrical Manufacturers Association (NEMA) established a joint committee whose task was to develop a standard for medical image communication. While the ability to acquire image data from various medical imaging devices is essential for the success of any

PACS system, it is not sufficient. The bits of information that make up the medical image must be associated with other information so that the acquisition modality unambiguously compiles the information the receiving system requires to fully use the images in question. The receiving system must be able not only to display, but also to analyze, process, reformat, and correlate the images it is dealing with. The successful PACS system must be interfaced to a radiology information system (RIS) and/or a hospital information system (HIS).

The data transferred among these different systems and the integrity of the same data are crucial for the functioning for the medical facility as a whole and the ED in particular. Medical imaging devices must accept key patient data and study identification information, associate this information with specific sets of images, and transmit both the image sets and the associated information to storage devices. To meet these requirements, there must be a universally accepted image format and a common communication protocol between the manufacturers. Since medical facilities often utilize equipment from a number of manufacturers, the manufacturers must agree to the standards described to allow a "plug and play" networking environment.[1]

The initial efforts of the ACR-NEMA committee resulted in the publication of the ACR-NEMA digital communication standard 300-1985.[2] This standard defined a point-to-point communication protocol, a standard set of command messages, and an agreed-upon data dictionary for image communication. It was based on a 16-bit parallel interface and was implemented by several vendors at that time. Based on the initial work with this standard, ACR-NEMA 300-1988 was published.[3] The new document, based on a 50-pin interface, was not extremely successful for several reasons. For example, it did not conform to the standard widely used in the communications industry, namely the seven-layered International Standards Organization (ISO) open-systems interconnections reference model for communications services.[4] Furthermore it was limited to point-to-point connections and contained a number of ambiguities, making it difficult for vendors to construct compatible implementations. It was immediately recognized that a third version of the ACR-NEMA standard would have to be written.

The third version of the standard, the Digital Imaging and Communications in Medicine (DICOM) standard,[5] established some degree of independence from the standards body and allowed international collaboration. DICOM is a multiple-part document that specifies (1) ISO-compliant protocol, (2) an industry standard protocol stack (TCP/IP), (3) an application layer support for both basic image communication and higher level functions and (4) an object-oriented data model.[6] DICOM was designed for a networked environment and therefore addresses an institutional or facility-wide need for image display and transmission. Version 3 of the DICOM standard, released for ballot by the ACR and NEMA in September 1993, is close to acceptance at the present time. Since 1992, the Radiological Society of North America (RSNA) has demonstrated the feasibility and functionality of the proposed standard at its annual meeting, held in Chicago. It is believed that most vendors of medical imaging and PACS equipment are complying with the DICOM standard in anticipation of its acceptance by the medical community. As the standard is incorporated by manufacturers, radiology workstations will be able to transmit and receive images and accompanying data within one facility or among many facilities geographically removed from one another: Once such hardware and software have been fully implemented, the present barriers due to proprietary equipment and networks will collapse.

The development of the DICOM standard and its acceptance by equipment manufacturers is the key to development of PACS systems. For PACS to be accepted in limited environments such as the ED, or in broader environments such as hospitals, certain functional requirements must be met. These include reliability, speed of retrieval and display, ease of use, productivity, and upgradability.[7] For years these functions of image and information management have been fulfilled, to greater or lesser degrees, by traditional radiology file rooms. The existence of PACS systems virtually eliminates the issues of access to and availability of imaging information so prevalent with traditional file rooms. Several types of system have evolved to meet these requirements. The development of these systems was driven by the application of the technology, not the technology itself. This continues to be the case as PACS is more widely implemented.

Acquisition and Display Systems

Systems have been designed as archival and review systems that basically operate by means of a frame-grabbing technology. These systems capture an analog image from an independent source, digitize it to 8 bits, and allow internal review of this material. These systems, which allow fast image acquisition with little duplication of technologist efforts, offer applicability to multivendor and multimodality environments, fast retrieval times, and image display in the original format.[8] Frame-grabbing systems have only two major limitations. Because the data are acquired at 8 bits, the ability to window and level (i.e., to change brightness and contrast) is lost. Second, storage at 8 bits in a converted format precludes three-dimensional reconstruction and data handling. Despite these limitations, frame-grabbing subsystems have met the requirements for electronic management of US, primary diagnosis in US, and secondary review in CT and MRI. Such systems clearly are not adequate for primary diagnosis of conventional x-ray images or primary diagnosis of CT and MRI images. These requirements, however, can be met by fully digital systems.[7]

Technology has now evolved for adequate networking, routing of data, and data transmission. Typically, dedicated image networks are required because of the large size of the individual files being transferred. Most data currently are transmitted in a noncompressed format. As lossless compression develops and becomes a reality, file size may decrease to the point of making shared networks possible.

The existence of the imaging data in a fully digital format allows a multitude of pre- and postprocessing features to be employed. In addition to standard corrections of window and level, image orientation, reordering of images, image adaptation, and remeasurement are possibilities. Studies have shown that in the PACS environment, up to 80% of images may require preprocessing before they are ready for review.[9] The required preprocessing functions included at a minimum correct orientation and a reasonable lookup table for display. With only these tools available, greater than 90% of the studies can be viewed. Processing functions such as reverse tables and edge enhancement, while generally not considered to be necessary, are highly desirable and tend to increase confidence in the diagnoses they support.

Display monitors come in a large variety of sizes and resolutions. It is imperative that the display monitor be chosen to reflect the functionality for which it is intended. As one might expect, increasing degrees of display resolution are tied to a logarithmic increase in the cost of the monitors. While high resolution, 2000-line monitors are required for primary diagnosis of chest and bone radiographs, lower resolution (1000-line) images are generally acceptable for use in consultation and review of images. The intensity of the monitor must be sufficient to prevent eye fatigue; luminance above 40 foot-lambert is adequate for low resolution monitors; substantial increases in brightness are required for higher resolution monitors (i.e., those with pixel numbers >2000). It has been suggested that low resolution monitors with high brightness levels may have diagnostic advantages over higher resolution monitors with lower brightness. Monitor brightness is also related to observer sensitivity to flicker. For most diagnostic applications with moderate brightness monitors, 60 Hz noninterlaced displays are acceptable. At luminescence above 50 foot-lambert, frame rates in excess of 72 per second are required.[10]

Many studies have been done to determine the resolution required for primary interpretation on CRT monitors. Some subtle abnormalities are detected with less accuracy in high resolution systems than in conventional film–screen systems. However, certain abnormalities, which depend primarily on contrast differences for detection, may be detected with greater accuracy when high resolution equipment is used than when recorded on conventional films. For most applications, a 1024-pixel monitor appears to be adequate. This certainly appears to be true for primary diagnosis of digital subtraction angiography, US, CT, MRI, and many projection radiography exams including bedside chest radiography. Investigation is still under way to determine whether the currently available high resolution technology (2048 pixel × 2536 pixel) is adequate for mammographic diagnosis and the detection of subtle bone fractures.[9]

Radiologists and clinicians have become accustomed to viewing multiple images simultaneously in CT, US, and MRI studies. Reproduction of this environment electronically is difficult and many be prohibitive from a cost standpoint. Rapid sequential viewing (ciné mode) of such studies on a limited number of monitors has successfully competed with simultaneous viewing in some studies.[10] Ciné mode viewing may thus be considered an acceptable alternative.

Digital Radiography

While PACS hardware, software, and network technology have advanced substantially, digital acquisition of conventional radiographic images has been slow to develop. Technology has been available for many years to convert analog radiographic film to a digital format through a laser scanning process. While this does accomplish digital conversion without significant information loss, it is a time-consuming process that can add up to 2 minutes per film cycle. When multiple films are taken on an individual patient, considerable time is added to the diagnostic cycle for each patient. Once converted, however, the data can be digitally viewed on an existing network at multiple sites by multiple clinicians. This feature also eliminates the major problem of film loss in the ED setting. The time trade-off is unacceptable in most busy EDs.

Computed radiography systems were initially developed for bedside chest radiography and have been in clinical use for at least 8 years. In such systems, a digital cassette replaces the standard film–screen cassette. Once exposed by x-rays, the cassette is "read" by a laser scanner in a special processing apparatus. Interfaces have been developed which link such systems to the radiology information system and reduce the need for duplicate data entry. Such systems have been successfully employed in the ICU setting for portable chest work and have been shown to have accuracies similar to those obtained with conventional film–screen radiography.[11] The small loss of resolution is more than compensated for by gains made in contrast resolution and postprocessing capabilities. However, the systems remain relatively slow, and the images are generally converted to analog output and printed by laser imager on conventional x-ray film rather than being read primarily on a monitor.

The systems just described have not had a major impact in the emergency department for several reasons. The time from the initiation of the x-ray to the delivery of the completed product remains relatively long and in fact is usually longer than that required for conventional film–screen radiography. Additionally, the algorithms that would allow the application of this technology to other ED settings (i.e., nonchest) have not been developed and/ or tested. While computed radiography has been used for screening abdominal/pelvic radioimages in trauma settings, its applicability in extremity radiography for the detection of fractures has not been clinically tested.

The technology necessary for the direct digital capture of fluoroscopic images has been in use clinically in the form of digital subtraction radiography. Again, system limitations in terms of resolution, cost, and size exist and somewhat limit the usefulness of this type of technology in the ED setting. However, extension of this technology to conventional radiographic imaging has been an area of intense research and development.

Recently, thin-film transistors (TFTs) and photoelectric diodes have appeared, designed for use in photoelectronic imaging devices. The initial development involved the use of small-area, flat panel, amorphous silicon imaging arrays, which are solid state and self-scanning. The amorphous silicon digital imager described by Antonuk et al.[12] has a format of 512 pixels × 560 pixels, a pixel-to-pixel pitch of 450 μm and an area of 230 mm × 252 mm. In this size format, examination of a small body part such as a hand is possible. A light-emitting x-ray converter such as a fluorescent screen remains an integral part of the imaging system. The light interacts with a sensor panel composed of the TFTs and photodiodes. The sensor panel converts the incident light to a charge in each photodiode. Charge can be stored during the acquisition, rapidly read out pixel by pixel in a digital format, and readily converted to a gray scale image using conventional hardware and software. The 450 μm pixel pitch (distance between center of adjacent photodiodes) corresponds to a resolution of 1.1 line pairs per millimeter.

While the spatial resolution of these flat panel imaging arrays is less than that of conventional currently available film images, the quality of the overall array is quite good. The contrast sensitivity is comparable to that obtained from conventional technology, and anatomic landmarks are well demonstrated. In phantom experiments, pathology can be recognized readily. Currently, development and evaluation of higher resolution arrays with a 1536 pixel × 1920 pixel format at a 127 μm pitch is under way.[12] This system exists on a flat panel substrate that is only 1 mm thick and would thus lend itself to packaging in a standard film–screen cassette arrangement. Such a device could be readily utilized in fluoroscopic equipment in the future. The single drawback in this configuration is the need to use a light-emitting screen. In comparison to direct x-ray capture, screen use imposes a finite limitation on resolution (Fig. 5.1).

The amorphous silicon TFT array used in conjunction with photodiodes is a first attempt to bridge the gap between conventional radiographic secondary laser scanning of cassettes and direct digital image capture. Two major limitations remain in terms of sptatial resolution and the need for conversion of x-ray data to light by means of a phosphorescent screen. Even though the amorphous silicon detector arrays are a giant step forward, the

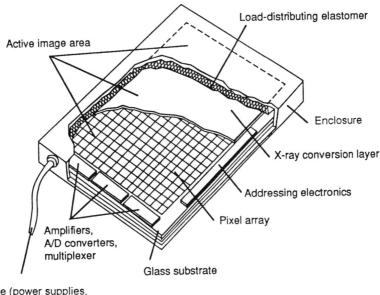

Load-distributing elastomer

Active image area

Enclosure

X-ray conversion layer

Addressing electronics

Pixel array

Amplifiers,
A/D converters,
multiplexer

Glass substrate

Cable (power supplies,
data transfer, control signals)

FIGURE 5.1. Schematic illustration of a selenium TFT and photodiode direct radiography detector. (Reprinted from Lee DL, Cheung LK, Jeromin LS. A new digital detector for projection radiography. *SPIE Proc*, vol. 2432, © 1995.

missing element for a filmless x-ray department and therefore a filmless ED x-ray department remains a suitable detector for projection radiography— that is, a device that can be used like conventional film–screen cassettes. Key requirements in the development of such a detector are (1) compatibility with existing x-ray equipment, (2) image quality and patient dose comparable to or better than those of competing film–screen combinations, and (3) competitiveness in cost per image with film–screen systems. Several computed radiography systems are commercially available and have achieved image quality and patient dose comparable to those obtainable with the older technology. However, the high capital cost and limited resolution potential of these dedicated systems have prevented their broad application. Meeting or exceeding all three of the requirements just stated has been a formidable challenge.

A direct digital detector for projection radiography has been developed and demonstrated.[13] This device employs TFT arrays in conjunction with photodiodes. Selenium is used as the x-ray photo conductor, and the necessity for x-ray-to-light conversion is completely eliminated (Fig. 5.2). Resolution in this device is limited only by pixel size, and a pitch as small as

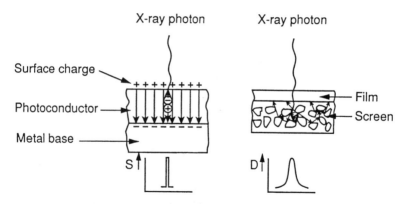

Figure 5.2. The interaction of x-ray photons with the photoconductor or film–screen results in a characteristic footprint. Shape and width of the footprint influence the lower limit of obtainable resolution. Notice that the "footprint" obtained from the photoconductor is narrower than that from the film–screen system. (Reprinted from Lee DL, Cheung LK, Jeromin LS. A new digital detector for projection radiography. *SPIE Proc,* vol. 2432, © 1995.)

139 μm has been achieved, resulting in line-pair resolution comparable to that obtained with film–screen combinations (Fig. 5.3). The detectors and TFT arrays have been able to achieve increased size as a direct result of huge investments made in the active matrix liquid crystal display technology by the flat panel display industry, as most widely employed in laptop computers. This technology has allowed the bonding together of several independent panels to achieve prototypes comparable in size to the standard 14 × 17 in. film commonly used in clinical settings.

This system was demonstrated at the RSNA meeting in Chicago in November 1995 and will soon be undergoing beta site evaluation at several large teaching institutions throughout the country. These TFT arrays demonstrate an excellent x-ray sensitivity and may actually allow a modest decrease in x-ray dosage compared to standard film–screen systems. In addition, because they are digital, they have a wide dynamic range and a broad latitude. This feature will dramatically decrease the need for repeating exams because of exposure errors. Spatial resolution, as already mentioned, is comparable to commercially available film–screen systems. Even in the highly demanding area of bone radiology, trabecular detail and overall contrast and gray scale have allowed the diagnosis of subtle fractures from soft panel readings. These devices promise to be economical and should be easily retrofitted into existing x-ray equipment and tables. Modifications for use as a portable capture device should be readily accomplished.

Exposure is electronically read out over a period of 2 to 3 seconds, and an image is available for review on a video display within 5 seconds of the exposure. The image data can then be manipulated (i.e., windowed, leveled, and subjected to postprocessing algorithms). For data processing, the system can utilize a commercially available PC with 32 megabytes of RAM. The device and resulting image are completely DICOM 3 compliant and thus will be readily incorporated into existing imaging networks. The last hurdle in terms of conventional image capture has almost been overcome, and selenium TFT arrays should be commercially available in the near future. At that point, fully functional networks incorporating MRI, CT, US, digital angiography, the techniques of nuclear medicine, and direct digital

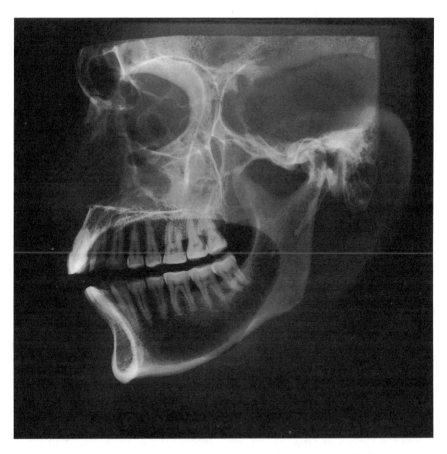

FIGURE 5.3. X-ray image of a mandibular phantom obtained using the selenium-based direct digital system. Note the excellent detail seen in the osseous trabeculae and in the teeth. Contrast resolution is excellent as well.

radiography will become a reality. Once instituted on a widespread basis, these networks should have a significant impact on productivity and patient management.

Looking to the future, long- and short-term storage devices and compression algorithms for digital data must be developed before a truly electronic radiographic record can be realized. While much progress has been made, considerable work, particularly in the area of lossless compression, remains. When the necessary advances have been accomplished, long- and short-term storage devices utilizing optical and magneto-optical disks or digital tape drive technology will be feasible.

A major limitation in current systems is the relatively long retrieval time required for single images, and particularly for the larger image sets used in CT, US, and MRI. Reloading of a single image frame from storage device to active network can require up to 15 seconds. Some of the time constraints can be overcome by "prefetching" of images for scheduled patients in a disbursed network configuration. This approach is obviously not applicable in the ED setting. Ultimately, the solution may lie in the development of personal image disks that patients maintain in their possession. These media could contain all or a significant part of each patient's recent imaging history and would undoubtedly include copies of the radiographic report appended to the individual studies.

Summary

Since the early 1980s, considerable progress has been made toward the realization of a completely electronic and filmless radiology department and emergency radiology subsection. Major advances have included the development of high speed, economical personal computers and file servers, the development of network technology and cable technology to allow high speed transfer of large data files, the development of the DICOM 3 standard for image transfer, the development of digital modalities such as CT, US, and MRI and, finally, the development of the technology allowing the direct digital capture of conventional radiographic images.

When implemented in the ED setting, a digital imaging network will significantly impact several areas of patient management. Imaging time per patient will be significantly decreased, because of the elimination of the needs for conventional film and film processing and because the number of repeat exams will be decreased as a result of the latitude of digital systems. The application of pre- and postprocessing algorithms will maintain if not improve the diagnostic quality of the images obtained. The images obtained from conventional radiography and cross-sectional modalities will be almost instantaneously available on a wide-area network in the radiology department and throughout the emergency department. This will facilitate the review of imaging studies by many health care providers, resulting in more efficient patient diagnosis and more rapid implementation of treatment algorithms.

References

1. Prior FW. Inforad: Informatics in radiology: Specifying DICOM compliance for modality interface. *Radiographics* 1993;13:1381–1388.
2. ACR-NEMA Committee. Digital Imaging and Communications. ACR-NEMA Standards Publication 300-1985. Washington, DC: National Electrical Manufacturers Association; 1985.
3. ACR-NEMA Committee. Digital Imaging and Communications. ACR-NEMA Standards Publication 300-1988. Washington, DC: National Electrical Manufacturers Association; 1988.
4. International Standards Organization. Information Processing Systems, Open Systems Interconnection Basic Reference Model. ISO 7498. New York: American National Standards Institute; 1984.
5. Horrii SC, Bidgood WD, Parisot CR, et al. *A Guide to the DICOM Standard.* Oak Brook, IL: Radiological Society of North America; 1994.
6. ACR-NEMA Committee. Digital Imaging and Communications in Medicine (DICOM) Part 2: Conformance. Final Draft for Letter Ballot, August 27, 1993. Washington, DC: National Electrical Manufacturers Association; 1993.
7. Gur D, Fuhrman CR, Thaete FL. Inforad: Computers for clinical practice and education in radiology: Requirements for PACS: User's perspective. *Radiographics* 1993;13:457–460.
8. Good WF, Burzik CM, Scanlon PF, et al. User-friendly electronic film library for digital imaging modalities. *Eur Radiol* 1992;2:494–495.
9. McNitt-Gray MF, Pietka E, Huang HK. Preprocessing functions for computed radiography images in a PACS environment. *Proc SPIE* 1992;1653:94–102.
10. Britton CA, Sumkin JH, Curtin HD, et al. Subjective perceptions of and attitudes toward primary interpretation of x-ray images. 1234:94–97.
11. Cox GG, Cook LT, McMillan JH, et al. Chest radiography: Comparison of high-resolution digital displays with conventional and digital film. *Radiology* 1990;176:771–776.
12. Antonuk LE, Yorkston J, Huang W, et al. A real-time, flat-panel, amorphous silicon, digital x-ray imager. *Radiographics* 1995;15:993–1000.
13. Lee DL, Cheung LK, Jeromin LS. A new digital detector for projection radiography. E.I. Du Pont de Nemours, Medical Products Department. Presented at the SPIE Meeting, 1995; San Diego, CA.

6
Intensive Care Unit

CARL A. SIRIO, G. DANIEL MARTICH, AND ANDREW B. PEITZMAN

Critical care units developed as an extension of postoperative recovery rooms and because of the dissemination of effective cardiac monitoring and respiratory support that is possible in such facilities. Intensive care units (ICUs) have proliferated worldwide with the expectation that they improve patient outcomes and overall quality of care by concentrating technology in the hospital environment. Admission is usually for intensive treatment of severe illnesses, for expectant monitoring to detect and prevent complications, or for concentrated nursing care unavailable in other hospital settings. These broad criteria for admission apply to patients who have sustained traumatic injury. Despite the presumed utility of critical care therapy, the clinical literature highlights conflicting evidence regarding its benefit. Consequently, consensus on the appropriate use of ICU resources does not exist. The growing capability to collect and analyze data for patients in the ICU may allow us to develop more meaningful criteria on which to base decisions regarding utilization and judgments regarding the effectiveness of critical care therapy for patients.

The ICU and Informatics

The ICU is an environment well suited to the automation and the dissemination of information technology, particularly given the large quantities of patient data routinely collected.

Effective use of the enhanced data management and computational power currently available must serve several functions if the bedside clinician and ICU managers are to be materially assisted in the care of injured patients. First, there must be ready access to information and manipulation of data, to permit caregivers to arrive at timely and effective decisions, and to decrease the likelihood of information overload. Second, the information derived must integrate data from multiple sources to produce integrated displays and reports. Finally, to facilitate clinical decision support, systems must evolve to utilize inferencing methods that allow detection of associations between various pieces of data that alert clinicians to serious or potentially life-threatening patterns of events.[1]

Developing an Integrated Patient Data Management System

Development and implementation of integrated patient data management systems for trauma patients in the ICU present significant challenges. These challenges can be classified to include issues related to data acquisition, data quality, data management and storage, data transfer, data presentation for clinical and research use, data confidentiality, and the costs and logistical support required to maintain and enhance operational systems.

Data Acquisition

Useful ICU systems must minimize the cost and work associated with inputting data. Interfaces with devices capable of generating digital signals, desirable because they reduce the labor associated with manual data collection, are potentially fraught with difficulty. Problems that must be overcome include proper identification of the digital signal linked with the patient in question. Further, given the potential for devices such as blood pressure transducers to generate extraneous signals, the quality of automatically collected data is not assured. Maintaining data flow can become problematic when patients must be moved for procedures or between the operating suite and the ICU. A standard language (HL7) has been developed to allow sharing of diverse sources on information in the hospital setting, but it has not been universally adopted by all suppliers of information system support to the health care industry. In addition, significant amounts of data continue to require manual input (e.g., patient physical examination findings).

Data Quality

Assuring the accuracy of analyzed and presented data is fundamental to maintaining confidence in any ICU information system. Several practical steps to minimize the perpetuation of erroneous data are suggested. These include frequent use of computerized data by caregivers to increase the likelihood that inaccuracies will be recognized; simple mechanisms to correct errors once identified; development of data filters to eliminate entry of data outside clinically credible limits; built-in redundancy and cross-checking of data between systems (e.g., pulse rates as determined by real-time ECG, arterial line, and pulse oximetry); minimization of hand entry of data;

and frequent generation of reports that require verification of the accuracy of data by responsible caregivers.

Data Management and Storage

A vast quantity of data is generated in the ICU, and the need to limit the amount stored presents a significant challenge. For what data points, and at what intervals, should data be captured and stored? The problems posed by these questions are under active investigation. This research is guided by the principle that the data collected and the intervals in which they are stored should be patterned to maximize the likelihood of capturing important physiologic change; such a pattern has a relationship to how data are collected and used clinically and should minimize inaccuracies generated by oversampling (e.g., minute-to-minute vital sign fluctuations).[2-4]

Few of the data collected in the ICU are actually utilized in patient care decision making. Before any algorithm is formalated for determining which data are captured, it should be determined which data are typically used by the patient care team when diagnostic and therapeutic decisions are made. For example, which of the multiple measured and derived data points regarding respiratory status in the intubated patient are used to make decisions regarding ventilatory support?[5-8] Furthermore, assuming certain data are required for bedside decisions, which of the data points collected need to be stored in long-term database archives? As the cost of data storage continues to diminish, it becomes ever more feasible to store all data. However, the volume of potentially available data may remain an encumbrance to users searching a database for future research or clinical questions.

Data Transfer

The ICU clinician and trauma researcher must have easily retrievable data if computer-stored data are to be of value. This requires that a system be established to allow uniform coding of data points.[9-11] Further, there is a growing need to standardize coding such that information can be shared across computer platforms with different operating systems. To date, our ability to utilize large amounts of information for multi-institutional research has been significantly hindered by our inability to easily transfer data between hospital information systems.[11-13]

Data Presentation and System Support: Critical Care Information System (CCIS)

An institutional decision to provide comprehensive CCIS support requires a multidisciplinary organizational and management approach. The components of this integrated structure must include representatives of the medical staff, nursing staff, and hospital administrative staff, as well as a dedicated technical support staff, including a team of system engineers responsible on a 24-hour basis for system hardware and software, programming, configuration, and system support.

Importantly, a CCIS must be configured and managed from the perspective of the clinicians responsible for patient care. This approach helps assure the clinical utility of a system once implemented and creates an environment in which customization of presented information can be solicited and incorporated into the system with relative ease. This factor is particularly important in the management of trauma patients whose care often becomes the responsibility of multiple clinical services. In these instances, data and information requirements may demand specific functional capabilities through the use of system macros and subroutines.[14]

A well-integrated CCIS should be directed toward synthesizing several, if not all, of the following characteristics: point-of-care electronic charting, menu-driven notes, interface with patient bedside biophysiological monitors to capture vital sign data, interface with the laboratory information system, management of medication administration and interface with pharmacy information systems, interfaces with ventilators, intravenous pumps, and other devices, and interfaces with risk adjustment and severity of illness tools.[14]

To facilitate use by busy clinicians, a CCIS should be designed to accommodate an individual workstation for each ICU bed. Additional workstations should be available at nurses' and physicians' work areas and attending physicians' offices. For ease of use, applications should utilize mouse-driven graphical user interfaces, "point and click" functional capability, user-configurable and context-sensitive pull-down menus, multiple integrated screens, and features that promote user training.

A well-designed CCIS will allow clinical uses that are varied and practically unlimited while assuring appropriate confidentiality of sensitive patient information. Data can be retrieved and entered at any workstation by any authorized caregiver. The CCIS workstation can serve as the focal point of daily rounds in conjunction with appropriate examination of the patient. Correlation between patient findings and stored information is facilitated by a CCIS that utilizes individual bedside workstations. With well-designed computerized flowsheets, a user can evaluate vital signs, laboratory data, ventilatory support settings and associated blood gases, intravenous infusion rates, medications, and nursing notes. The bedside workstation architecture represents a distributed computing environment providing extensive processing power and speed.

CCIS data storage allows for ease of access to patient data throughout the ICU and subsequent hospital and posthospital discharge periods. Importantly, the storage of information in databases utilizing database tools such as Structured Query Language (SQL) facilitates export of data to systems designed for patient research or decision support.

Outcome Measurements

There are four advantages to improved and accurate severity of illness data in predictive models of outcome in trauma management generated by computer-based software applications. This capacity to provide risk-adjusted severity data utilizing validated predictive models is becoming widely available in the ICU. Each of these plays a role in improving the delivery of health care.

First, these models allow physicians to focus aggressive intervention on individuals most likely to benefit. As resources become constrained, physicians must decide which clinical problems are most likely to benefit from ICU care. There is growing consensus in the medical community that objective measures of illness should play a part in ICU admission and discharge decision making.[15]

Second, physicians caring for critically ill patients are often faced with decisions regarding the withdrawal or limitation of therapy. Prognostic information, accurately predicting outcome, can serve as an adjunct to these difficult decisions. Recent work suggests that appropriately validated risk adjustment tools for predicting short- and long-term benefit from ICU care can be used constructively to improve clinical decision making in this area.[16,17] Third, prognostic systems relying on large databases can facilitate the assessment of new technologies and allow for comparative analysis with established modes of therapy. Clinical therapies using accurate and reliable pretreatment risk stratification controls can improve the value of the information derived from trials for trauma patients by reducing the amount of unexplained variation in patient risk. Fourth, the benefit of precise prognostic estimates allows for ready comparison of the performance between ICUs and institutions. This is particularly important in supporting and maintaining regionalized trauma systems.

Current efforts to assess severity of illness for trauma patients center around either trauma-specific prognostic indices, such as TRISS, or general risk adjustment tools such as APACHE. While TRISS has been widely validated in trauma patients, it is designed primarily for documenting unexpected outcomes with respect to prehospital and emergency department care, not ICU care. Further, although widely utilized, TRISS has not been widely incorporated into existing critical care systems. TRISS and APACHE offer examples of the role of risk adjustment in the care of trauma patients and the interplay of the information required to compute these severity scores with trauma informatics in the intensive care unit.

TRISS

Measures developed to assess trauma injury severity were fostered by several overlapping phenomena. These included the growing regionalization of trauma care, federal attention and funding coincident with the recognition of trauma as a major epidemic, and the proliferation of ICUs.[18]

TRISS is a representative example of an index widely validated in the care of trauma patients. TRISS was designed primarily for documenting, tracking, and evaluating outcomes from trauma care by means of a system based on patients' anatomic, physiologic, and age characteristics. Anatomic scoring is based on injury severity score, and physiologic status is quantified using the Revised Trauma Score (RTS).[19] Calibrated to patients during assessment in the emergency department, TRISS has not been calibrated to a representative population admitted to the ICU from a diverse group of hospitals following traumatic injury. Further, being limited to trauma, TRISS does not provide ready comparisons of outcomes within or across institutions for patients suffering from other diverse maladies. Lastly, TRISS outcome predictions are limited to assessing hospital mortality following injury and are not designed to serve as bedside adjuncts to decision making.

Nevertheless, institutional performance and quality assurance reports regarding trauma care frequently rely on TRISS to risk-adjust patient severity of illness. PC-based software products are available to facilitate the collection and analysis of TRISS data. These products have typically been stand-alone programs and are limited by their inability to interface with ICU and hospital information systems.

ICU Decision Making

Decisions in critical care center around three distinct topical areas: triage, patient-specific diagnostic and therapeutic determinations, and the choice of an overall strategy for the organization, management, and structure of ICU delivery.

Triage decisions have an overall impact on the quality of care before, during, and after admission to the ICU. Diagnostic and therapeutic judgments, as well as the organization and structure of the ICU, affect the quality of care during the period of time spent in the ICU.

Within the context of providing high caliber critical care for trauma patients, the value of assessing severity of illness for clinical decision making, quality assessment, and utilization review has been ever more apparent to the clinician at the bedside, especially when the information is provided in real time and can be used to assist ongoing patient care. The capability of prognostic systems to provide this information is becoming a reality as efforts to develop CCIS and to automate prognostic and severity indices have borne fruit. As databases continue to expand, the predictive ability of these systems may be improved and refined.

APACHE III

Until recently there has not existed a national benchmark for comparison of outcomes across a wide variety of diseases in critical care. APACHE III allows for the establishment of a national, mortality-based performance assessment standard for all hospitals with more than 200 beds.

The APACHE III prognostic system consists of two major components. The first is an APACHE III score, which can provide initial risk stratification for severely ill patients within defined homogeneous patient groups, such as traumatic injury. The second element is the APACHE III predictive equation, which uses the APACHE III score and the national reference database, containing disease categories and treatment location prior to ICU location, to produce patient-specific hospital mortality and other important outcome risk estimates. The overall predictive accuracy of the first-day APACHE III equation is such that for 95% of patients, a risk estimate within 3% of those observed is produced within 24 hours of ICU admission. Similar accuracy can be obtained over subsequent ICU days by means of independently generated and validated regression models developed from the reference database.[20-22]

Data from the APACHE III normative database have been incorporated into the APACHE III Management System (System). This is a commercial system designed to provide real-time clinical information to physicians, nurses, and other clinical staff to support the effective treatment and management of critically ill medical and trauma patients. Using the APACHE III database, the System may enhance triage decision making while patients are being considered for admission to and discharge from the ICU by allowing clinicians to more effectively develop rigorous criteria on which to base these decisions. Furthermore, with the capability to produce daily updated predictions of risk and mortality, as well as other clinically relevant end points, the System allows for objective insights into the impact of ongoing diagnostic and therapeutic decisions. These capabilities will enhance the quality assurance and utilization review activities within an institution and allow for the effective comparison of institutions providing care for traumatically injured patients.

Also, to facilitate utilization review and quality assessment activities, the System provides physicians and other interested managers summary data of an outcome from trauma services over time. Importantly, this capability allows for improved short- and long-term planning and evaluation of trauma services. In addition, it will help institutions meet the requirements

for monitoring care posed by the external review agencies that pro-
vide certification to trauma centers, as well as such organization as the
Joint Commission for the Accreditation of Healthcare Organizations
(JCAHO).

To provide these capabilities as well as several not specifically discussed
in this chapter, the System is designed around several distinct modules.
These include data entry, clinical decision support, utilization management,
system administration, and ad hoc reporting. The two modules most relevant to clinical practice in an ICU providing care to trauma patients are
the clinical decision support module and the utilization management
module.

Clinical decision support provides risk predictions for individual patients
and displays detailed information for selected patients. The information
provided by this module is designed to facilitate discussion regarding triage
decision making and ongoing diagnostic and treatment evaluations. The
utilization management module allows the user's ICU and hospital performance to be compared directly against the reference database. This database can be updated over time to keep the normative predictions current.
The data provided in this module are integral to the System's ability to
provide valuable information for both quality assurance and utilization
review activities.

The System is based on a UNIX operating system and is currently ported
to Sun MicroSystems Sparc Station. The System, which can be linked with
multiple workstations and utilizes a graphic laser printer, runs an Oracle
relational database management software and uses the X Window System
for a graphical user interface. The System is designed to be electronically
interfaced with clinical laboratory information systems and the hospital's
admission, discharge, and transfer systems. Importantly, interface capability to other ICU information systems is available, enhancing the capabilities
of CCIS for the clinician.

Decision Support in the Care of Trauma Patients

The use of comprehensive decision support systems within the ICU and
for the care of trauma patients remains a laudable goal.[23-26] To date, many
decision support systems have been designed as expert systems to address a single issue, such as diagnosis utilizing a decision modeling algorithm.
Currently there are few comprehensive and well-designed systems
that integrate hospital information and decision support programs for the
ICU.

The HELP system, designed at LDS Hospital in Salt Lake City, Utah, is
the most frequently cited example of a comprehensive decision support
system for extensive use within the ICU. The HELP system is designed to
provide clinical *alerts* regarding time-critical decisions, data assimilation to

facilitate *interpretation* of information, clinical *assistance*, utilizing predictive information to improve decision making, computerized analysis of clinical decisions to *critique* the appropriateness of decision making, diagnostic decision support utilizing available clinical data, and ICU *management support*. At present, systems analogous to the HELP system are not widely available for use in ICUs.

Conclusion

Huge amounts of data are available to the clinician in the ICU. Our challenge is organize these data in ways that allow the clinician to synthesize information and improved medical and management decision making. Development of comprehensive information systems that support a broad array of decision-making needs is imperative if informatics is to play a significant role in the management of trauma patients admitted to the ICU.

For computer-stored data to be helpful, they must be easily retrieved. It is important that the data be in a standard format useful to clinicians, researchers, and administrators so they can be used for a variety of purposes. The proof of the success of a medical informatics system is its clinical acceptance and the use of the system for patient care.

As demonstrated by examples discussed in this chapter, institutions are taking increased advantage of informatics in the care of traumatically injured ICU patients.[27] However, advances in the application of computer technology in the care of the critically ill are likely to be incremental for the foreseeable future, as significant hurdles remain in the integration of existing and near-future technologies into the ICU.

References

1. Clemmer TP, Gardner RM, Shabot MM. Medical informatics and decision support systems in the intensive care unit: state of the art. In: Shabot MM, Gardner RM, eds. *Decision Support Systems in Critical Care.* New York: Springer-Verlag 1994;1:3–24.
2. Gravenstein JS, DeVries A Jr, Beneken JFW. Sampling intervals of clinical monitoring variables during anesthesia. *J Clin Monit* 1989;5:17–21.
3. Bradshaw KE, Gardner RM, Clemmer TP, Orme JF Jr, Thomas F, West BJ. Physician decision-making—Evaluation of data used in a computerized ICU. *Int J Clin Monit Comput* 1984;1:81–91.
4. Knaus WA, Wagner DP, Lynn J. Short-term mortality predictions for critically ill hospitalized adults: Science and ethics. *Science* 1991;254:389–394.
5. Gardner RM, Hawley WH, East TD, Oniki T, Young HFW. Real time data acquisition: Experience with the Medical Information BUS (MIB). *Surg Clin North Am Comput* 1991;15:813–817.
6. East TD, Yang W, Tariq H, Gardner RM. The IEEE Medical Information Bus of respiratory care. *Crit Care Med* 1989;17:580.

7. Sittig DF, Gardner RM, Morris AH, Wallace CJ. Clinical evaluation of computer-based, respiratory care algorithms. *Int J Clin Monit Comput* 1990;7:177–185.
8. Sittig DF, Gardner RM, Pace NL, Morris AH, Beck E. Computerized management of patient care in a complex, controlled clinical trial in the intensive care unit. *Comp Methods Prog Biomed* 1989;30:77–84.
9. McDonald CJ. The search for national standards for medical data exchange. *MD Comput* 1984;1:3–4.
10. McDonald CJ. Interchange standards revisited. *MD Comput* 1990;7:72–74.
11. McDonald CJ, Hammond WE. Standard formats for electronic transfer of clinical data. *Ann Intern Med* 1989;110:333–335. Editorial.
12. Agency for Health Care Policy and Research. Report to Congress: The feasibility of linking research-related data bases to federal and non-federal medical administrative data bases. AHCPR Publ. No. 91-003. Rockville, MD: AHCPR; April 1993.
13. Agency for Health Care Policy and Research. Report to Congress: Progress of research on outcomes of health care services and procedures. AHCPR Publ. No. 91-004. Rockville, MD: AHCPR; May 1991.
14. Martich GD, Hazy JC, Hravnak M, Dale B, Stein KL. Case study: A critical care information system. *Proc Healthcare Comput* 1994;205–216.
15. Society of Critical Care Medicine Ethics Committee. Consensus statement on the triage of critically ill patients. *JAMA* 1994;271:1200–1203.
16. Knaus WA, Harrell FE, Lynn J, et al. The SUPPORT prognostic model objective estimates of survival for seriously ill hospitalized adults. Study to understand prognoses and preferences for outcomes and risks of treatments. *Ann Intern Med* 1995;122:191–203.
17. Esserman L, Belkora J, Lenert L. Potentially ineffective care: A new outcome to assess the limits of critical care. *JAMA* 1995;274:1544–1551.
18. MacKenzie EJ. Injury severity scales: Overview and directions for future research. *Am J Emerg Med* 1984;2:537–549.
19. Boyd C, Tolson MA, Copes WS. Evaluating trauma care: The TRISS method. *J Trauma* 1987;27:370–378.
20. Knaus WA, Wagner DP, Draper EA, et al. The APACHE III Prognostic System: Risk prediction of hospital mortality for critically ill hospitalized adults. *Chest* 1991;6:1619–1636.
21. Knaus WA, Wagner DP, Zimmerman JE, Draper EA. Variations in mortality and length of stay in intensive care units. *Ann Intern Med* 1993;118:753–761.
22. Wagner DP, Knaus WA, Harrell FE, Zimmerman JE, Watts C. Daily prognostic estimates for critically ill adults in intensive care units: Results from a prospective, multicenter, inception cohort analysis. *Crit Care Med* 1994;22:1359–1372.
23. Pryor TA, Gardner RM, Clayton PD, Warner HR. The HELP System. *J Med Sys* 1983;7:87–101.
24. Prokosch HU, Pryor TA. Intelligent data acquisition in order entry programs. *Proceedings of the Twelfth Annual Symposium of Computer Applications in Medical Care*, 1988;454–458.
25. Bradshaw KE, Gardner RM, Pryor TA. Development of a computerized laboratory alerting system. *Comput Biomed Res* 1989;6:575–587.

26. Pryor TA, Clayton PD, Haug PJ, Wigertz O. Design of a knowledge driven HIS. *Proceedings of Eleventh Annual Symposium on Computer Applications in Medical Care*, 1987;60–63.
27. Gardner RM, Shabot MM. Computerized ICU data management: Pitfalls and promises. *Int J Clin Monit Comput* 1990;7:99–105.

7
Rehabilitation Informatics

Jeffrey S. Hecht, Alfred G. Kaye, Gregory D. Powell, and Carl P. Granger

Aspects of Rehabilitation Practice Relevant to Information Systems

Ideally, rehabilitation should begin early in the continuum of trauma care. Rehabilitative issues include avoiding preventable problems such as decubiti, deep venous thrombosis, and contractures. Thus, there can be rehabilitative issues addressed by emergency medical technicians, emergency room physicians and nurses, transporters to and from radiology, and nurses and physicians in the intensive care unit and later on the hospital floor. Rehabilitation is most effective when started early—not waiting until the patient is in a "rehabilitation center."

Rehabilitation has three major principles:

1. Secondary disability should be prevented. For example, the primary condition may be a fall from a motorcycle with brachial plexus injury to the left arm and bilateral tibia fractures. Contributing factors to disability in this patient include the decubitus ulcer incurred as the patient is transported on a hard stretcher to and from radiology, the hypoalbuminemia and nutritional deficit that occur as the patient is fed intravenously between the various operations to salvage the legs and remains catabolic for 3 weeks, and the superimposed causalgia that develops in the area of the plexopathy.

2. The disability caused by the primary medical condition impairment may be only a fraction of the primary total disability. Examples include the patient who becomes depressed and is therefore unwilling to participate in therapy, the family problems that accompany unrealistic expectations that a patient will be independent at discharge when the medical condition makes it impossible (e.g., when involvement of three limbs makes a patient dependent on transfers—at least until he is able to bear weight on two limbs), and a premorbid superimposed problem such as an underlying alcohol addiction that, unrecognized, leads to delirium tremens in the ICU setting—and to recurrent injury if ignored and untreated.

3. Diagnosis of disability is not equal to the diagnosis of disease.

The third principle deserves some clarification. For example, a patient presents to the emergency department following a motor vehicle wreck with a Glasgow Coma Score (GCS) of 12 and left hemiplegia. He is found to have a small right subdural hematoma, not large enough to require evacuation. The diagnosis of disease is clear: traumatic brain injury with right subdural hematoma. The diagnosis of disability requires more questions and more time. Is the patient right- or left-handed? What was his vocation or avocation? If he is a laborer who enjoys playing the violin, a diagnosis of disability is severe. If he is a right-handed accountant who collects coins, the diagnosis of disability can be less threatening.

Of course, our example requires a knowledge of the time course of improvement and other associated factors. Does the patient show rapid improvement in thinking skills, such as memory, attention, and judgment, or is there a prolonged posttraumatic amnesia? How is the functioning of new, intermediate, and remote memory affected? Is there an associated left homonymous hemianopsia? Left hemisensory deficit? Or left hemi-incoordination as the paresis resolves? Does the patient have a nondominant parietal lobe syndrome that will impair judgment and ability to return to work even if there is a full return of motor functions? Are there emotional changes such as flat affect or temper and violent outbursts? In what state does the patient live? Early seizures may have no relation to late seizures. However, some states do not allow driving for 2 years following a seizure. This restriction can present a marked vocational disability even though the patient may otherwise have an excellent recovery. All these issues impact on rehabilitation.

The wide differences in disability in patients assigned the same medical diagnosis have made it impossible for the Health Care Financing Administration (HCFA) to assign diagnostic related groups (DRGs) to rehabilitation. HCFA found traditional medical conditions similar enough to be grouped into DRGs and set fixed payments for each group with variation based on outlines. Despite many years, it has proven impossible to apply this billing method to rehabilitation. Primarily, this is because there is so much variation. To some extent, this is a limitation based on the nomenclature—that is, the disability groups are not well enough defined. This is being studied and may change in the future.

In many settings, formal therapies begin with an order for physical therapy to begin work on range of motion, or occupational therapy to develop splints to help prevent contractures. In some cases, these services are initiated or coordinated by a specialist in physical medicine and rehabilitation (physiatrist) or a rehabilitation nurse/case manager. The services of other disciplines such as speech pathology and psychology can be initiated by these specialists individually or as a multidisciplinary group. All these disciplines have the need to document the following in the medical record: their evaluations, their goals, and their ongoing progress notes, as well as units of treatment for billing purposes. The therapist generally may initiate treatment in the ICU setting and then expand the program when the patient is on the floor and better able to participate in therapies.

In the most progressive settings, the multidisciplinary team of treating professionals and social services meets with the team leader to comment on progress and address interdisciplinary goals. For example, therapists may intermittently accompany physicians on rounds, or they may have one or more formal meetings weekly. There is an additional documentation need for therapists at discharge—to document the total progress achieved and functional status at discharge. There may be a need to document family and patient education regarding the nature of head injury, spinal cord injury, and other disabilities. There is the need to document counseling interventions. Appropriate documentation of therapeutic gains in the chart can facilitate transfer to the next level of care outside the hospital setting—whether it be intensive inpatient rehabilitation, skilled nursing facility care, intermediate nursing facility care, or home health care.

Following discharge from the trauma center, there is the need to document appropriateness of personnel involved in transfer, sharing of information, and results of intervention in the next setting. There are computer systems available to list nursing therapy goals for home health and to comment on progress toward achieving those goals. In general, however, physicians may find them to be filled with jargon and woefully lacking in useful information. In general, there is a lack of sharing good information with the treating physician who must recertify the need for home health services. Therapists should note progress made from one session to another, but they tend to list the functional status at that point. Skilled nursing facility services are generally better in this regard, but performance among institutions varies. Some centers have well-developed information systems and the ability to document progress. Others require much searching through daily progress notes to determine what if anything has been achieved.

Inpatient rehabilitation centers are more thorough in documentation. The Commission on Accreditation of Rehabilitation Facilities (CARF) was established in 1966 by a multidisciplinary group of professionals and institutions interested in inpatient rehabilitation. The goal was to develop standards for the field, and the emphasis has been on program evaluation as well as quality assurance. There are a variety of tools for measuring progress at different levels of complexity. Some are nationally accepted. There is the need for therapists, physicians, and nurses, with some systems, to document the level of function at admission and then serially on a weekly or biweekly basis. A final assessment is made at discharge. There is the requirement for an assessment of function after discharge as well.

Rehabilitation: A Historical Perspective

Since its early years, rehabilitation medicine has been in the forefront of medical fields interested in informatics. This is due to several factors.

1. There was the need to prove to other physicians that the techniques of this new field made a difference. Therefore, data on outcomes of increasing complexity were felt to be required.

2. The emphasis on outcomes research led to ever more complex systems to measure the results of rehabilitation on individual patients and patient populations.

3. A multidisciplinary team approach generated large amounts of information that had to be compiled in a form more readily digestible than traditional hospital records.

4. It become ever more apparent that communication problems interfered with good rehabilitation. For this reason, data-banks were generated to facilitate interaction among members of the treatment team.

5. Data on functional assessment instruments, efficiency of treatment, and later utilization review and quality assurance became increasingly important to managers of rehabilitation units and to physicians responsible for quality in a rehabilitation program. Increasingly sophisticated tools were needed to generate meaningful information.

6. As cost pressures mounted, it became more important to reduce the time in producing reports. Therefore, tools were developed to produce reports more quickly and with greater consistency between reports. This trend, which is particularly manifest in the areas of psychology that call for neuropsychiatric assessments using standardized tools, has carried over, as well, to such areas as speech pathology and occupational therapy.

7. Computers were used as tools in training of cognitive functions in areas of psychology/behavioral medicine, speech pathology, and occupational therapy, to address issues of cognitive retraining therapies. Journals and new companies were created to meet the information demands of this growing field. Measurement of outcomes and results of treatment were in turn required to produce evidence of successful outcomes of therapeutic interventions for third-party payers.

Initially recognized as a medical specialty in 1947 with the establishment of the American Board of Physical Medicine and Rehabilitation, PM&R (physiatry) already had a track record of outcome research demonstrating benefit. The prolific writer and pioneer of rehabilitation, Howard A. Rusk had demonstrated to the U.S. Army and to physicians throughout the world through numerous papers that active rehabilitation is superior to passive convalescence in restoring soldiers to duty. In his writings, Dr. Rusk separated medical interventions into three phases:

preventive medicine
surgery and curative medicine
rehabilitation[1]

Outcomes research led to the recognition of a phase "between the bed and the job" when active rehabilitation programs can lead to greater functional outcomes.

In the early years, proponents of rehabilitation were somewhat evangelical because of the resistance of many physicians to changing old habits of prolonged convalescence following abdominal surgery or myocardial infarction. Where studies could be carried out, this was done, and data were generated. New tools evolved to measure these functional changes. These were called tools for functional assessment.

Functional assessment is a method of describing limitations and disabilities in order to measure an individual's use of the skills needed to perform tasks relative to daily living, leisure activities, vocational pursuits, and social interactions. For a given functional assessment, selected descriptive diagnosis performance social roles are used.[2] A variety of tools arose, including the Barthel Index,[3] the Katz ADL Scale,[4] and the Kenny Scale[5] (from the Sister Kenny Rehabilitation Institute in Minnesota). The PULSES Profile was developed to look at a wide variety of factors affecting rehabilitation outcome, including social issues.[6]

In 1976 Granger and others introduced the long-range evaluation system to measure functional assessment in a more sophisticated manner.[7] This tool combines features of the PULSES Profile, the Barthel Index, and social features that were a component of the Escrow Profile.[8] Granger's system later led to development of a more readily accessible tool that is now accepted by a majority of rehabilitation centers: the Functional Independence Measure Scale (FIMS). This tool is discussed in more detail later.

Harvey and Jellinek developed a tool called the Patient Evaluation Conference System (PECS), which measures a patient's functional level with 79 items on seven-point rating scales in 14 areas. This system is used in over 30 facilities.[9] There is also an outcome tool looking at the level of independent living and productivity in adults.[10]

Using the scales, it is clear that there is a trade-off between having enough information to show changes in an individual patient versus having so much information that it becomes a cumbersome tool and difficult to use to assess progress in a population. The latter application (i.e., assessing progress in a population) was the reason for growth of the FIMS system, which is easy to use and well supported by a national data base in Buffalo, New York. In addition, FIMS has been shown to have high reliability between different testers; that is, it is high in test–retest reliability and intercoder reliability.[11]

Some systems have so many detailed areas of assessment that any single area may not add much to the total outcome picture. For example, the Texas Institute of Rehabilitation and Research (TIRR) in Houston had a tool that measured some 113 items. One study showed that some of these items correlated so well with others that reporting one was sufficient. One such case consisted of the items for brushing one's teeth and washing one's face. A person who could do one task could do the other as well.

Data collection forms, required for the use of functional assessment tools, include descriptive checklists that provide the clinician with clear definitions of each skill level. The forms are designed to make entry into a computer relatively easy. Mutually exclusive definitions are developed for the descriptive criteria to reduce ambiguity in rating. Educational materials are developed in workshops conducted regularly to teach the uniform criteria to users of the FIMS system.

Data from various patients can be compiled so that certain populations (e.g., victims of multiple trauma, head injury, or spinal cord injury) can be studied as a group. One may look at the entire group of trauma patients or split them as much as needed. The more one knows about this field, the more one tends to be a splitter, because different outcomes are expected for different levels of injury. For example, patients with C-5 complete quadriplegia can be expected, with adaptations, to brush their teeth and wash their faces and propel electric wheelchairs, but they will always need physical help for transfer skills and most bed mobility, as well as high level bladder and bowel care and advanced activities of daily living (ADLs) such as lower extremity dressing. Patients with C-7 quadriplegia often can be basically independent in transfers and mobility at the wheelchair level but have limited endurance and respiratory capacity. Only the most unhealthy of patients with low paraplegia are not able to be independent in mobility and self-care skills at the wheelchair level. To lump all spinal cord–injured patients together is to neglect these differences.

When the Commission on Accreditation of Rehabilitation Facilities was established over 30 years ago, its mission was to improve the quality of services to people with disabilities, to develop and maintain state-of-the-art standards for use by organizations to improve their performance, and to share information among programs. Since its early years, CARF has emphasized the need for a program evaluation system. In fact, the commission developed a "special policy on program evaluation,"* which is summarized in its *Standards Manual* as follows:

The organization needs a continuous program evaluation system as a means of identifying and evaluating the outcomes and results of the services it provides to people against pre-established goals. At the same time, the Commission recognizes that this can be accomplished only with a substantial and demonstrated commitment on the part of the organization over an extended period of time. Such a commitment must originate at the highest level of the organization.

CARF says that the system must include a description of the following:

A. The goal of the program.
B. The types of people services.
C. The services provided in the program.
D. The objectives to be achieved and the measures of accomplishment.

---

*This phrase and the following excerpts and shorter quotations from the CARF *Manual* are found in Reference 12.

E. The methods for collecting, processing, reporting and disseminating evaluation data.

For a program to be accredited, the commission requires a program evaluation system to be in progress and a management report generated within 6 months. The *Standards Manual* notes that "Program evaluation should be used to measure progress in relation to the overall program goals. . . . [and] Program evaluation information should be integrated into the organization's decision making at all levels." This is an area that readily lends itself to informatics. Indeed, the manual calls for a review and evaluation, at least annually, of the relationship between the needs of the person served and the services being provided, a report to be supplied by the organization's staff and governing authorities. The evaluation tool, the manual continues, must "measure outcomes of programs and services—A, B. Include all persons served or representative sample. C. Regularly measure the progress of persons served in relation to program goals. D. Evaluated post-discharge information."

The FIMS system meets the basic needs of program evaluation under CARF by providing scales that show change in functional status from admission to discharge. It is hoped that future tools will allow the measurement of functional status at times after discharge from the rehabilitation center or perhaps at fixed points following the initial onset of trauma. For assessing a pediatric trauma program, for example, the American College of Surgeons requires use of Wee-FIMS, a version of FIMS modified to apply to nonadult patients. Wee-FIMS scores are then required at 6 and 12 months after onset of the initial trauma. It is hoped that at some point the same program evaluation tool can be used by both trauma programs and rehabilitation programs so that their respective data can be integrated into a common system.

Unfortunately, that type of system is not readily available in the 1990s. In fact, most rehabilitation programs struggle to meet their specific needs in a matrix circumscribed by restrictions of the large mainframes and standard hospital management information systems. Information systems currently include demographics and are moving toward developing severity indexes. However, their tools for measuring outcomes do not approach the level of sophistication required in measuring outcomes under rehabilitation. Such tools are proposed by Williamson in *Assessing and Improving Health Care Outcomes*.[13] The Glasgow Outcome Scale for head injury is likewise grossly inadequate because it does not have enough steps between the normal or asymptomatic state and death. It is too gross a tool—using it is like trying to cut diamonds with a chain saw. Unfortunately, rehabilitation centers have been forced to develop their own systems.

Rehabilitation units associated with larger, acute care hospitals have had to develop their own software packages to integrate with the hospital's mainframe if they wish to develop a database that includes information from both systems without having to cue in all the demographic information a second time. Some centers (e.g., Parkview Regional Rehabilitation Center, Fort Wayne, IN) have been creative enough to go on to use these systems to develop reporting tools for the therapist. It is possible to develop such sophisticated management information tools as a means of tracking how many hours of therapy are provided by individual therapists and recording these data in graph form against projected targets. Likewise, outcomes of patients grouped by therapists or screening physicians may be used to give feedback to the treatment team or individuals on the team as to how their results stack up against those of their peers for cases of the same type. This can be a helpful educational tool. Rehabilitation centers that are parts of larger chains have the benefit of using tools developed for those systems. They are often supplemented by a cadre of computer programmers who help with data entry.

Unfortunately, one system does not communicate with another. The national FIMS databank operates with its own separate computer system and does not integrate into other hospital management information systems. Although FIMS is flexible enough to allow measurement of certain data, it does not allow the integration of management information tools such as those noted above, report generator tools, and long-term follow-up data points. Also, the financial data entered comprise basic charge data that are not adjusted for the discounts actually given by a facility, nor is FIMS able to account for true costs generated by the facility. Rather, the system includes a limited number of data points and does not cover the full spectrum of rehabilitation. It tends to show the greatest changes with patients in the midrange of their rehabilitation and very slow changes for the more severely disabled and those at the higher range of function. For example, a patient with a 5-month-old head injury who is walking, talking, and unemployed and on the welfare rolls has the same FIMS score as a person with the same medical status who is gainfully employed and a taxpayer. Such crudeness may not make much difference in that functional assessment tool, but it matters greatly to society. Certain postacute rehabilitation programs that address the transition to social and community integration and ultimately to work might have great success in meeting their goals but show no change under the FIMS system.

Perhaps this a problem with our definition of "health care" overall. Generally we are defining health care as just Rusk's second phase and some of the early parts of the third phase. The greatest reductions in cost to society may lie at the extremes—preventing disease and returning the unemployed to gainful employment or reducing their level of dependence on the system.

What is the economic cost of dependency? In the United States in 1990, over 10 million people received disability payments for assistance in maintaining themselves. This represented 7% of the gross national product, and it went to disability payments made to approximately 5% of the population.

Among the working population of disabled individuals, disability payments were nearly four times medical program expenditures. For disabled persons, even disregarding the loss of earned income, the costs of maintenance represented approximately 75% of the direct cost of disability.

In the 1980s, most state Medicaid expenditures went to nursing home care—far higher than the expenditures for acute hospital care and physician services. The state of Minnesota, for example, spent 53% of these monies for nursing homes, 14% for inpatient hospitals, and 6% for physician services. Reducing the extent of dependence can therefore be cost effective.

Impairment, Disability and Handicap: Definitions, Significance, and Challenges in Measurement

Before a measurement tool for the assessment of rehabilitation outcome can be developed, we must establish what is to be measured. Various tools have been developed that grade a patient based on various clinical, historical, or performance-rated criteria.[14,15] These tools, however, perform in different ways. The primary categories in which a rehabilitation candidate is measured are impairment-based and handicap-based. To determine which scale is the more practical, we must first understand their definitions.

An impairment is defined by the World Health Organization as "any loss or abnormality of psychological, physiological, or anatomical structure or function."* It is the limitations posed to the patient by the body's response to the pathologic problem. For example, a patient who has suffered a T-12 spinal cord injury may exhibit loss of sensation below the T-12 dermatome, weakness or paralysis of muscles below the T-12 myotome, and hip flexion contractures from heterotopic ossification. Loss of sensation, weakness, and loss of range of motion are all considered impairments. While this information can be useful, it does not define function to an extent adequate to allow for the measurement of outcome.

The World Health Organization defines *disability* as "Any restriction or lack resulting from an impairment of ability to perform an activity in the manner or within the range considered normal for a human being." This definition adds a new dimension to the evaluation of a patient. A particular diagnosis (e.g., T-12 paraplegia) does not define the disability. Indeed, many factors contribute to the disability encountered by a particular patient, including impairments, motivation, and such preexisting problems as pain, obesity, or substance abuse. In our example of T-12 paraplegia, inability to walk would be the patient's primary disability, resulting from sensory

---

* References 16 and 17 contain the World Health Organization definitions quoted in this section.

loss, weakness, and loss of range of motion. This category of criteria provides the best standardized means of evaluation of function.

The World Health Organization defines *handicap* as "a disadvantage for a given individual resulting from an impairment or a disability that limits or prevents the fulfillment of a role that is normal (depending on the age, sex, and social and cultural factors) for that individual." In other words, this is a societally imposed restriction. For example, if our T-12 paraplegic was unable to keep a job in a second-floor office because the building did not have an elevator, the patient's condition would be considered a handicap. These situations become so variable regionally that functional outcome measurement often is impractical.

Sometimes the terms blur. As observed in the book *Disability in America*, "Disability is an issue that affects every individual, community, neighborhood, and family in the United States. It is more than a medical issue; it is a costly social, public health, and moral issue."[18]

Disability is growing in tandem with the growth of trauma itself. For every 100 injuries in a given year, 9 years are lost. This is a particular problem in young adults, who commonly incur mobility limitations, such as those due to spinal cord injuries, orthopedic impairments, and paralysis.

The per-person economic costs associated with spinal cord injury (SCI) and traumatic brain injury (TBI) are among the highest for injury-related diagnoses.

Studies published in the last 15 years reported incident rates of traumatic brain injury in the United States ranging from a low of 180 per 100,000 people in the San Diego, California, area, to a high of 367 per 100,000 in the Chicago area. The National Head and Spinal Cord Injury survey estimates a rate of 200 hospitalizations per 100,000 people per year. Applying this to the 70-year expected life span for Americans, an individual could be said to have a greater than 10% chance of suffering a head injury.

The acute severity of traumatic brain injury has traditionally been measured using the Glasgow Coma Scale (GCS), a 13-point scale ranging from 3 to 15. Although GCS is highly correlated with survival, it poorly predicts long-term quality of life.

While most individuals hospitalized for TBI are diagnosed as having a mild, uncomplicated closed head injury, recent evidence suggests that one third of those employed prior to injury do not return to work within 3 months and that over 50% have persistent headaches or difficulties with memory. The true economic impact of these injuries is yet to be calculated.

Each year 70,000 to 90,000 individuals sustain moderate to severe head injuries that result in life-long potentially disabling conditions. Two thousand sustain injuries severe enough to result in a "persistent vegetative state." The National Head Injury Foundation describes this as the "silent epidemic." Yet because the sequelae are more neurobehavioral than physical, and because of representations in the media associating head injuries with quick full recovery, public expectations in this area are unrealistic. Contrary to the image of head injury portrayed on television shows, persons who suffer a severe head injury seldom return to work the next week with no residual deficits. In fact, a study by McKenzie in 1987 indicates that 88% did not return to work within 6 months and 71% had not returned to work within a year.

In recognition of the dearth of information on incidence, outcomes, and long-term function in patients with head and spinal cord injury, the Committee on the National Agenda for the Prevention of Disabilities recommended that the national health interview survey be expanded to include questions regarding the circumstances and cause of injury to help improve our knowledge of injury etiology. A comprehensive supplement on incidents, medical care, rehabilitation, and disability related to injury is strongly recommended.

Information from the National Hospital Discharge Survey (NHDS) is limited because of inconsistencies in use of the CM codes, in the ninth revision of the International Classification of Diseases (ICD-9) the lack of uniform coding of the external cause of injury, and the lack of functional diagnoses, making it impossible to determine patient's true impairment status.

The Committee on a National Agenda for the Prevention of Disabilities recommends that people who have potentially disabling injuries receive adequate acute care and rehabilitation:

Universal access to coordinated system of care that integrate treatment from the site of the injury through long-term community follow-up is recognized as essential for mitigating the short-term effects of SCI and TBI and for controlling the effects of long-term disabling conditions.[19]

The four basic elements of such a coordinated approach can be summarized as follows:

1. Emergency medical services (an acute medical/surgical care)
2. Acute (medical) rehabilitation
3. Psychosocial and vocational rehabilitative services
4. Life-long comprehensive follow-up

A system of care for TBI patients (Fig. 7.1) is just now evolving. Head injury is much more complicated than traumatic spinal cord injury in that presentations, outcomes, and sources of treatment vary so much.

Informatic systems that wish to convey a true picture of outcome in patients with traumatic brain injury will consider the neural behavior impairments that contribute to the greatest functional limitations of the traumatic brain injured. Rather than simple activities of daily living and motor deficits, these are harder to classify but more highly correlated with ultimate outcome. The ultimate goal of physical, psychosocial, and vocational reha-

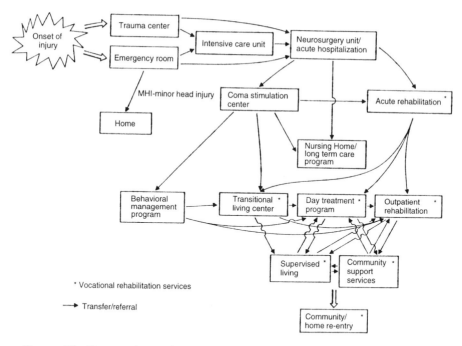

FIGURE 7.1. Care continuum in traumatic brain injury. Follow-up activity is needed to identify and treat potential sequelae in persons who initially require only outpatient treatment (see the box marked "Home"). (From JM Uomoto and A McLean, Care continuum in traumatic brain injury rehabilitation. *Rehabil Psychol* 1989;34(2):71–79.)

bilitation is community reintegration—that is, return to work, school, family, friends, and perhaps a new role in society. It is important that every stage of the coordinated system of care look ahead toward the next phase in efforts to minimize complications and facilitate the most effective rehabilitation.

It is obvious that the concepts of impairment, disability, and handicap complicate our ability to find appropriate functional measurement tools for trauma patients. An adequate understanding of the concepts, however, provides a foundation for critical examination of various measurement tools.

FIMS and Functional Assessment

Accountability for providing quality health care delivery is as important for medical rehabilitation as it is for the entire health care industry. The focus of physical medicine and rehabilitation is to improve the functional status of patients. Finding valid and reliable methods of assessing functional outcome is necessary to justify the value of rehabilitation.

Currently, the Health Care Financing Administration reviews quality for all Medicare recipients based on a case-by-case system known as the Peer Review Organization (PRO). According to Audet and Scott,[20] evidence that PROs improve the quality of health care is still lacking. These authors suggest that quality measures be reviewed at the local or institutional levels to provide more accurate and valid data on practice.

In the early 1980s, medical rehabilitation moved toward a facility-based model of program evaluation. This concept was premised by reviewing a set group of common elements that indicate functional status of the patient—thus bypassing the case-by-case methodology of the PRO system. Currently, HCFA appears to be moving toward a more continuous quality improvement and education orientation similar to that of medical rehabilitation for program evaluation through the Uniform Clinical Data Set (UCDS).

The Uniform Clinical Data Set will likely become the national database for Medicare's quality review program. This database took 5 years to develop and can accommodate up to 1800 clinical variables per patient case. The elements of the UCDS include patient identification, history and physical examination, laboratory results, diagnostics, surgical interventions, endoscopic procedures, therapeutic interventions, inpatient medications, recovery phase, discharge status, and discharge planning.

In today's environment of change in delivery to managed care networks and capitation, case-by-case review could become obsolete for performance evaluation measures. The move is toward facility-to-facility comparisons of functional outcomes. Contracts are established on the overall outcomes of functional performance in relation to cost and quality.

The term "functional assessment" refers to a method of appraising a person's abilities in an accepted environment. What fundamental skills are necessary to survive in a day-to-day existence? Individuals use a variety of skills to perform daily tasks such as self-care, leisure or avocational activities, and vocational activities. All involve some form of social, cognitive, and/or physical skills. The functional assessment measures these abilities and skills.

Many instruments have been developed over the last 30 years to measure the quality of medical rehabilitation outcomes. These include the Barthel Index,[3] the Index of Independence in Activities of Daily Living (Katz),[4] the Kenny Self-Care Evaluation,[5] the Level of Rehabilitation Scale (LORS), the LORS American Data System (LADS), the Patient Evaluation and Conference System (PECS),[9] the Pongee System Inc. Easter Seals System, Client Case Management, and Program Evaluation (I-PASS), and the Functional Independence Measure (FIM). The development of a good functional assessment tool requires a clear conceptual framework; valid,[21] reliable,[22] and relevant responses; an easy and logical format; a reasonable amount of time for execution; and the ability to forecast outcomes in a clear, concise, understandable, and timely manner. Rehabilitation professionals had no accepted standard of functional assessment with consistent terminology to communicate about disability until the 1980s, with direction from the Commission on Accreditation of Rehabilitation Facilities and the standards on program evaluation.

Currently, one of the largest nationally used functional assessments for medical rehabilitation is the Functional Independence Measure, managed by Uniform Data System for Medical Rehabilitation (UDSmr) located at the State University of New York in Buffalo.[23,24] The FIM was developed in 1984 to measure the functional outcomes for physical rehabilitation. Initial grant support came from such agencies and organizations as the American Congress of Rehabilitation Medicine, the American Academy of Physical Medicine and Rehabilitation, and the National Institute on Disability and Rehabilitation Research of the Department of Education. Carl Granger and Byron Hamilton were given charge as codirectors of the task force responsible for developing the desired uniform data system, the UDSmr.[25]

The theoretical basis for the FIM is that level of disability indicates burden of care. To be disabled entails a cost both to society and to the individual for the latter's lack of independence. These costs impact social and physical areas. Human and/or physical resources such as medical supplies, assistive devices, and/or attendants will be needed to help the disabled person approach or reach independence. Fundamentally, resources equate to time, money, and energy.

The FIM was developed as a minimum data set that would be appropriate only for key functional attributes of patients. The attributes (elements) are discipline free, acceptable to clinicians, administrators, and researchers. After examining 36 published and unpublished functional assessments, the task force identified elements and rating scales for the FIM. The items selected for the FIM assess self-care, sphincter control, transfers, locomotion, communication, and social cognition. The FIM rating scale measures the elements on a scale of 1 to 7 (1 = dependence; 7 = total independence). The rating scale is administered quickly and uniformly and demonstrates valid and reliable measures.

The FIM provides a tracking system of patients from admission to discharge and follow-up, with periodic update assessments to measure changes in patient performance. The FIM includes information on patient demographic characteristics, diagnostic groupings, impairment groups, length of inpatient rehabilitation stay, cost of stay, payer mix, and discharge placement, in addition to the functional outcome measures and trends. Subscribers of UDSmr receive reports quarterly during the calendar year.

The UDSmr continues to work on pilot, trial, and implementation studies as well as to upgrade the clinical and technical features of the FIM. Since 1988, subscribers of UDSmr have been able to submit data files of individual case records to a central database that currently has over 300,000 patient records for the United States. This information provides the opportunity to establish standards and trends on national and regional levels.

Currently, there are 470 inpatient medical rehabilitation facilities in the 49 states that have enrolled with UDSmr. UDSmr is international, in use in Japan, France, Canada, Portugal, Italy, Sweden, Germany, Spain, and Australia. Since 1988, over 200 workshops have been held, instructing over 6000 clinicians, program evaluation coordinators, and administrators.[26,27]

The Uniform Data Set for Medical Rehabilitation requires facilities wishing to subscribe to be credentialed. This process is twofold. First the facility undergoes training and testing to develop an acceptable level of rater reliability. Second, a technical review of the facility's data is performed to monitor the guidelines for technical adequacy. (The Guide for UDSmr is available from UDSmr[SM] Data Management Service, University at Buffalo, South Campus, 232 Parker Hall, 3435 Main Street, Buffalo, NY 14214; fax (716) 829-2076; (716) 829-2080; e-mail FIMNET@ UBVMS.CC.BUFFALO.EDU).

Figures 7.2 to 7.6 illustrate the FIM data for the year July 1, 1993 to June 30, 1994. These figures make use of the following abbreviations: SELCRE, self-care/ADLs; SPHNCT, sphincter control; TRANSF, transfers; LOCOM, locomotion (wheelchair or walking); COMMUN, communication skills; and SOCCOG, social, cognitive factors.

The FIM is computerized, and the software, called FIMware, is designed to run on an IBM-compatible 486 computer operating at a minimum speed of 25 MHz with a minimum of 4 megabytes of RAM (8 MB preferred), and a hard disk with a minimum of 5 MB of available storage up to 20 MB as the database expands. FIMware is written in Windows format with the ability to provide custom reports using spreadsheet programs such as Lotus, dBase, and Excel.

The USDmr FIMware Implementation and User Guide describes the systems benefits to subscribers as follows:

For clinicians:

  a tool for consistently assessing severity of disability;
  a way to monitor patient gains and outcome;
  key data for rehabilitation program evaluation and quality improvement activities;
  information for patient management and clinical team conferences
  national standards and normative data relating impairment and level of disability to the outcome of care;
  a resource for training;
  a resource for research.

For administrators:

  information for analyzing and monitoring the quality of care, program evaluation, and support of accreditation procedures;

  data for determining cost benefit ratio and effectiveness of rehabilitation care;
  a basis for predicting rehabilitation outcome and utilizing this information for establishing admission and discharge criteria, as well as referral to alternate appropriate services;

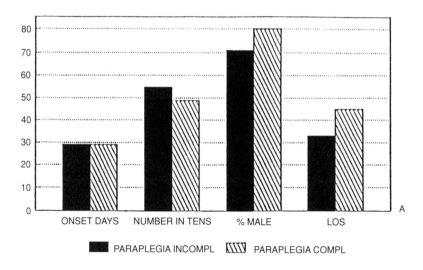

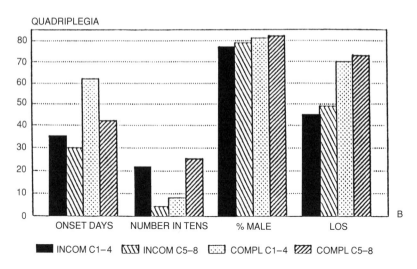

Figure 7.2. FIM data for spinal cord injury resulting in paraplegia (A) and quad-riplegia (B).

a potential basis for justifying payment of services;

a way to feed information back to care providers to facilitate clinical and administrative decision making and the development of policies and procedures which will improve the rehabilitation process.

Functional assessment measures may forecast trends and predict outcomes more closely as these instruments improve and better reflect the clinical and financial environment of physical medicine and rehabilitation. The use of functional assessment tools to hold medical rehabilitation as an

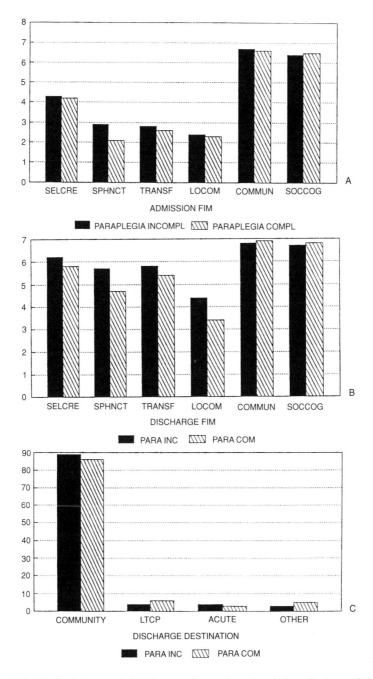

FIGURE 7.3. Marked changes in FIM scores from admission (A) to discharge (B) are noted in paraplegics undergoing comprehensive rehabilitation. (C) The majority are discharged home. SELCRE = self-care/ADLs; SPHNCT = sphincter control; TRANSF = transfers; LOCOM = locomotion/wheelchair or walking; COMMUN = communication skills; SOCCOG = social, cognitive factors. (From Uniform Data System, 1993.)

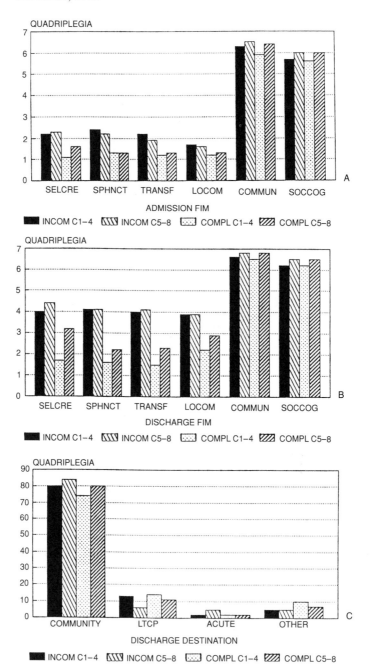

FIGURE 7.4. (A, B) Marked gains in function is seen in quadriplegics undergoing comprehensive rehabilitation as measured by FIMS. (C) Even high quadriplegics who enter specialized spinal care centers are discharged home over 75% of the time. (From Uniform Data System, 1993.)

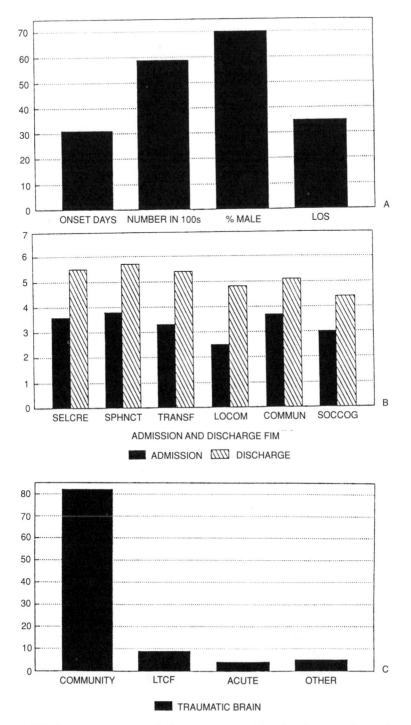

FIGURE 7.5. Severe traumatic brain injury demographics, showing gains from admission (A) to discharge (B) in FIMS scores, as well as discharge destination (C).

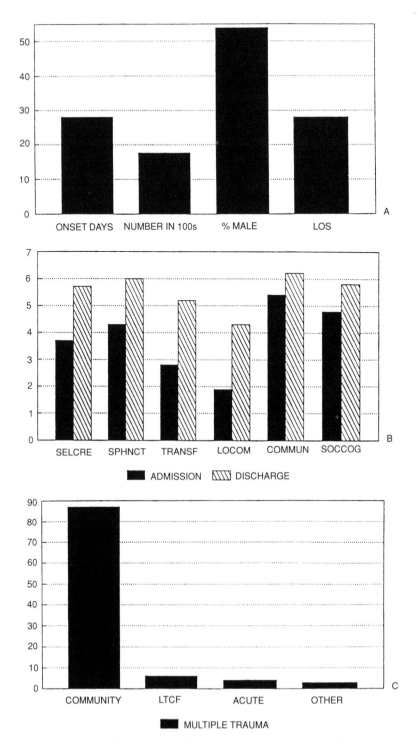

FIGURE 7.6. Severe multiple trauma demographics, showing gains from admission to rehabilitation (A) to discharge (B) as measured by FIMS scores and excellent outcomes in discharges to home (Uniform Data System, 1993).

TABLE 7.1. UDS national first admissions for brain dysfunction

	1990	1992	1993
Number of patients	1822	3367	5081
Males	69%	69%	69%
Females	31%	31%	31%
Mean age (years)	38	40	41
Mean onset (days)	37	34	31
Mean admissions FIM total	64	62.1	60.9
Median admissions FIM	64	63	62
Mean discharges FIM total	97.7	95.2	94.5
Mean discharges FIM	109	105	104
Mean length of stay (days)	46	40	36
FIM gain per week	5.3	5.8	6.5
Discharges to community	82%	83%	82%
Discharges to long-term care facility	7%	8%	9%
Discharges to acute care	5%	5%	5%

accountable and credible mode of health care delivery of service only enhances the need for medical rehabilitation. Functional assessment is the cornerstone of program evaluation, allowing comparison of the effectiveness and efficiency of medical rehabilitation to effect patients' transition from traumatized victims to functioning, integrated participants in society.

Some Data from the Fourth Annual Report of the Uniform Data System for Medical Rehabilitation

Tables 7.1 and 7.2 reflect the growth in medical rehabilitation hospitals and units participating in FIMS. From 1990 to 1993, more than twice as

TABLE 7.2. USD national first admissions for traumatic spinal cord injury dysfunction

	1990	1992	1993
Number of patients	904	1723	2655
Males	72%	73%	74%
Females	28%	27%	26%
Mean age (years)	43	42	42
Mean onset (days)	41	37	33
Mean admissions FIM total	64.1	65.3	65.7
Median admissions FIM	62	63	64
Median discharges FIM total	90.2	90.4	91.6
Mean discharges FIM	99	98	99
Mean length of stay (days)	51	45	43
FIM gain per week	3.6	3.9	4.2
Discharges to community	78%	82%	83%
Discharges to long-term care facility	7%	7%	6%
Discharges to acute care	6%	5%	6%

many hospitals participated in data submission, building information on three times as many patients as reported in 1993 than 3 years previously—about 127,000. Of these, the 5081 traumatic brain injury patients represent 4% and the 2655 spinal cord injury patients represent 2% of the total.

Commission on the Accreditation of Rehabilitation Facilities Standards

The ever-changing CARF standards* should be considered in the development of an information system. This body's requirements for program evaluation systems include the following:

A. Admission criteria. B. A listing of services offered. C. Measurable objectives. D. A specification of the time for which each measure is applied. E. Priority ranking and weighing of the objectives. F. Measures of effectiveness and safety. G. Measures of the satisfaction of the person served with the program.

The system should track and maintain at a minimum: A. Characteristics of persons served—e.g., diagnoses, functional limitations, types of disabilities. B. Services received. C. Dates of service—e.g., entrance/admission and exit/discharge. . . .

5. Program evaluation and management reports should reflect: A. Measures of effectiveness—e.g., benefits achieved by the person served. B. Measures of efficiency—e.g., time, cost, utilization, etc. C. Measures of the satisfaction of the person served with the program. D. Characteristics of persons served. E. Interpretation of results.

6. Information produced by the program evaluation system should be made available to appropriate levels of management on a timely basis. Such information should be used by management to discontinue, maintain or improve the program. A. The organization should have a means to determine when performance is less than acceptable. B. When performance falls below the acceptable level, the reason should be defined. C. Management should take action and improve program performance at an acceptable level. D. Follow-up and monitoring of corrective actions should be performed at specific times with the results documented.

7. There should be evidence of utilization of program evaluation information at all levels of the organization involving administrative functions—e.g., resource allocation, policy setting, long range planning, marketing, etc., and in programmatic functions—e.g., determining admission requirements, developing service delivery techniques, etc.

8. There should be an annual professional administrative review of the characteristics of the person served that includes: A. Consideration of the appropriateness of the intensity and type of service provided. B. Documentation as to whether changes are occurring in the service population which indicate the need for service modification or expansion.

---

*Excerpts from the CARF standards quoted in this section are from Reference 12.

9. Program evaluation information should be made available in an understandable fashion and should be communicated in a timely manner to the government authorities, personnel and the organizations and including persons served, purchasers of services, and supporters.

10. A mechanism should be maintained to provide for a continuous review of the adequacy of the program evaluation system. This mechanism should provide for: A. Formal review taking place on an annual basis. B. Personnel affected by the evaluation system having an opportunity to recommend or make modifications. C. An assessment of the systems success to increasing benefits, controlling or reducing program costs, and maintaining improving community support. D. A determination of the efficiency of the program evaluation system.

11. Results obtained from the program evaluation system should be integrated with a consumer-based planning process.

In the area of spinal cord injury programs, CARF recommends that the treatment plan be based on integrated interdisciplinary assessment; the following three areas should be included in the databank for such programs:

1. Pathological diagnoses (e.g., ICD 9-CM, American Spinal Injury Association classifications).
2. Impairments (e.g., American Spinal Injury Association Motor Index).
3. Functional limitations.

Other areas mentioned in the spinal cord injury program standards that lend themselves to the benefits of informatics include CARF's standards 2 and 4:

2. The program should be part of an acute hospital that is capable of caring for persons with neural trauma or should have a formalized relationship with such a hospital, along with demonstrated mutual consultive services beginning early post-trauma. The relationship should provide: A. An exchange of information. B. Inservice education. C. A sharing of common treatment protocol. D. Arrangement for transfer into the spinal cord injury unit.

4. Appropriate clinical information should be received prior to and at the time of transfer into the unit.

Informatics systems are used to access databanks in accordance with CARF standards 7 to 9.

7-A. Community integration services including supervised community excursions and provisions for overnight therapeutic passes. There should be referral to appropriate available community services such as independent living, recreation, home health services, education, vocational rehabilitation, transportation, etc.

7-B. Recommendations regarding environmental modification—e.g., home, school, or work site modification. It is important that patients be followed long term, and informatic systems can be used to help with keeping in touch with patients and then following up through clinics to meet other standards: . . .

7-C. Follow up for health maintenance.

8. There should be an organized program of follow up to maintain and/or to improve health status following discharge.

9. There should be written plan of follow up care. The spinal cord injury program should provide its own follow up care for those persons remaining in its service area. Arrangements for follow up care should be made for persons who leave the programs to graphic service area. The follow up plan should provide: A. Referral and forwarding of medical information to a designated physician in other appropriate medical organizations and community services. B. Follow up appointments with the spinal cord injury unit and/or a designated physician. C. Therapy programs, equipment checks, neurological evaluations. D. Psychological, social and community reintegration services. E. Designation of an individual to be responsible for coordination of the person's follow up plan.

One should obtain the latest edition of CARF standards which are updated annually. Even now, the commission plans to modify its standards through the third millenium to reflect changes in health care provision—while respecting the dignity and individuality of persons served.

It would be helpful to document the effects of educational programs on the community through documentation of contacts as well. Such information also could serve as a tool to assess a level of understanding in the spinal cord injury community to meet CARF standard 11: "Quality organization should demonstrate efforts to educate the community in the prevention of spinal cord injuries."

Educational programs also lend themselves to benefits of informatics. Some programs use individual computer-based teaching modules to supplement or replace individual classes and textbooks. This practice meets standards for the following "formally organized and mandatory participation in program for the person served/family and spinal cord injury education." The program above should provide for, but not be limited to, education regarding:

(1) Bladder management. (2) Bowel management. (3) Equipment care and community resources for repair. (4) Instructions and medications. (5) The need for follow up medical care and how to access it. (6) The need for attendance [sic] and how to secure and manage them. (7) Nutrition. (8) Pulmonary care. (9) Skin care. (10) Substance abuse. (11) Use of leisure time.

Some of the issues are the same in traumatic brain injury. Many programs find computer systems to be helpful to maintain policy and procedures and upgrade them with changes in standards in health care regulations.

Issues in Quality Management of Rehabilitation for the Physician Executive

Rehabilitation informatics is a key tool for management by the physician executive employed in a modern health care organization. The trade-off between the cost and quality of medical care is an area that requires both medical and management decisions for each patient. Thus, as described by

Leland Kaiser, the physician executive is an "interfaced professional."* Observing that most of the problems in contemporary health care fall on this interface between medicine and management, he points out: The health care field is moving toward integrated data bases and data base management. Hard facts will replace opinions as health organizations upgrade their management information systems. The physician executive needs data concerning the impact of physician practice patterns on the financial welfare of the organization. He can use these data to modify physician behavior.

The computer is critical in making financial decisions. Kaiser continues:

Everything in the organization reduces to economics. If you understand how the money flows in an organization, you understand most of the organization's dynamics. If you understand how physicians are reimbursed for their services, you can explain a lot of the variance in their practice patterns and professional behavior. You must be alert to the financial impact of all the decisions you make.

Issues include cost accounting, pricing, taxes, financial management, budgeting, and investments. Again, Kaiser elaborates:

Changes in reimbursement policy and procedure are a constant problem for all health provider organizations. The physician executive needs to examine the impact of such changes on physician behavior, organization response, costs and quality outcomes, and organizational repositioning in the market place.

Hard data are critical to bring about modification of physician behavior and to facilitate organizational change in response to changes in reimbursement policy and procedure. Informatics is critical to affect cost and quality outcomes and to effect organizational repositioning in the market place.

The trade-off of cost versus quality is an issue that has been widely debated. Although JCAHO has addressed standards of care issues, there is currently no universally accepted ranking of the elements of quality. Klint and Long listed the following as "major elements of a health care quality matrix":

(1) Physician—Technical (input). Capabilities and characteristics of physicians are reflected by training, board certification, continuing education, liability history, medical records and level of activity (numbers of procedures performed/diagnoses made). (2) Hospital—Technical (input). Licenses, accreditation, and other official evaluations of institutional competence such as JCAHO findings, university affiliation, currency of technology, nursing staffing ratios, level of activity (numbers of procedures performed) and liability history. (3) Physician—Art (process). "Art of care." Characteristics of physicians are reflected by peer review findings, rapport with patients, availability, and listening and instructing capacities. (4) Hospital—Subjective (process). Hospital characteristics including staff attitudes, service orientation, appearance, ambience, guest amenities, reputation and empathy. (5)

---

*This phrase, and the three longer quotations that follow, are from Reference 28.

Continuity of care (process). The degree to which a comprehensive spectrum of health care services exist, including services such as education, preadmission planning, discharge planning and follow up care as appropriate. . . . (6) Mortality (outcome). (7) Morbidity (outcome). Occurrence of complications or other outcomes that are less than ideal including hospital-acquired infections, repeated procedures, length of stay if more than two standard deviations above the mean. Or, if discharged, delayed returns to desirable functional outcome, or readmissions for the same diagnosis. (8) Customer satisfaction (outcome), evaluations (both subjective and objective) of patient's care from the perspective of lay party such as patients, families, employers and other purchasers.[29]

Another definition of quality is provided by Rodriguez:

Produces optimal improvement in the patient's physiological status, physical function, and emotional intellectual performance, consistent with the best interest of the patient. (2) Emphasizes the promotion of health, the prevention of disease or disability, and the early detection and treatment of such conditions. (3) Seeks to achieve the informed cooperation and participation of the patient in the care process and in decisions concerning that process. (4) Is based on accepted principles of medical science and the proficient use of appropriate technological and professional resources. (5) Is provided with sensitivity to the stress and anxiety that illnesses can generate and with concern for the patient's overall welfare. . . . (6) Makes sufficient use of the available technology and other health systems resources needed to achieved the desired treatment goal. (7) Is sufficiently documented in the patient's medical record to enable continuity of care and peer evaluation.[30]

Unfortunately, the tools do not yet exist in the field of rehabilitation for measuring the severity of conditions within a diagnosis. The tools developed for acute care severity standards, as discussed by Iezzoni,[31] do not truly apply to rehabilitation.

Medical quality management programs have been developed to facilitate the ability to monitor rehabilitation.[32] Hospital governing bodies delegate the responsibility for implementation of medical quality management programs in the organized medical staff. This work often falls to the medical executive committee and the informatics system. Insofar as these functions are relevant to implementation, their scope includes (1) monitoring the evaluation of the quality and appropriateness of patient care provided by all individuals, (2) drug usage evaluation, (3) medical record review, (4) pharmacy and therapeutics functions, (5) infection control, (6) hospital safety, and (7) utilization review.

It is also critical that data obtained from the medical quality management program (MQMP) be appropriately transmitted between committees and ultimately to the chief operating officer, the medical executive committee, and the institutional board. According to one published set of guidelines:

Data collected as part of the MQMP must be analyzed and evaluated by individuals who are in positions to make informed judgements. Nothing is served by having data entered into a "black hole." The critical locus for information use is the clinical department, usually defined as the active staff of that department. Information from the MQMP must be shared with the active staff so that corrective action can be taken as necessary and the results monitored.[33]

Information must go to clinical departments, therapy directors, appropriate diagnostic program committees, the chief operating officer, and the medical executive committee. Because rehabilitation functions by putting a multidisciplinary team together that often addresses a particular clinical condition such as spinal cord injury or traumatic brain injury, the chain of information flow usually differs from that seen in acute care hospitals. In the more sophisticated organizations, therapists have professional responsibilities within their departments that fall into the purview of utilization review and quality assurance; in addition, they have outcome and process responsibilities within their diagnostic programs (that fall under review by quality assurance and program evaluation).

Like acute care hospitals, rehabilitation centers are involved with developing clinical/critical pathways to deal with particular diagnoses in a more standardized fashion. These evolved from efforts by the American Medical Association, the Rand Corporation, and the Health Care Financing Administration to establish "clinical practice parameters" or "practice guidelines." It should be recognized that while there is a range of possible clinical management strategies to diagnose and treat different patient conditions, falling outside the standards of care could be defined as deviant or negligent—suggesting evidence of failure to comply with acceptable standards of care if the behavior of such a physician or therapist "fell clearly outside the boundaries of the parameters without any forthcoming justification for that deviation."[34] On the other hand, following such guidelines may actually decrease exposures.

Quality assessment monitors vary from hospital to hospital and from institution to institution among rehabilitation centers. There is no standardized program that is as widely used as that to monitor program evaluations such as the FIMS. Programs remain fairly labor intensive at this juncture.

Retrospective chart review is not easy. Indeed, it is

a laborious and tedious process. . . . People performing it are prone to make transcription errors and to overlook key data. One of the great appeals of computer-based medical records is their potential ability to facilitate the chart-review process. Such records obviate the need to retrieve hard copy charts; instead, researchers can use the computer based data retrieval and analysis techniques to do most of the work (finding relevant patients, locating pertinent data, and formatting the information for statistical analyses).[35]

A nice discussion by a physician of the use of databases to measure health care quality is available.[36]

Pediatrics

Despite the limitations, rehabilitative outcome measures are fast becoming part of the standard outcome measuring tools in trauma. The National Institute on Disability and Rehabilitation Research (NIDRR) has been involved with the development of the National Pediatric Trauma Registry. This form has nine sections: (1) patient identification, (2) demographics in injury, (3) scene of injury, (4) admission to participating trauma center, (5) injury severity assessment on admission, (6) trauma center management, (7) trauma center discharge, (8) anatomic diagnoses, and (9) therapeutic and diagnostic procedures at time of injury. Section 7 includes the length of time children have deficits in vision, hearing, speech, self-feeding, bathing, dressing, walking, cognition, and behavior. Outcome measurements include the FIM adaptation to children, Wee-FIM. The areas include self-care (feeding, grooming, bathing, dressing, and toileting), sphincter control (bladder and bowel), mobility in terms of transfers (bed to chair, toilet, tub), and locomotion (walking or in wheelchair and on stairs), communication (comprehension and expression), and social cognition (social interaction, problem solving, memory).

Participation in the registry is a requirement for designation as a specialized pediatric trauma center through the American College of Surgeons. Pediatric trauma centers are asked to get follow-up Wee-FIM scores on patients 6 and 12 months after the initial trauma.

The Uniform Data System for Medical Rehabilitation launched the Wee-FIM subscriber service on April 1, 1994. This direct adaptation of the functional independence measure for adults uses the same 18 items with a seven-level rating scale, but takes the pediatric patient's growth and development into account. Version 4.0 is available in both in- and outpatient formats and for follow-up after inpatient stays. Follow-up assessments using the Wee-FIM are recommended 80 to 180 days postdischarge. Over the course of the hospitalization, interim assessments can be performed at the facility's discretion. Version 4.0—Outpatient will be used to track changes in function abilities over long periods of time in school-based and even home-care settings. Information on Wee-FIM can be obtained by contacting Susan Brun, Director of Wee-FIM Services, UDS Data Management Service, 232 Parker Hall, 3435 Main Street, Buffalo, New York 14214 [phone: (716) 829-2076].

Informatics in Spinal Cord Injury Rehabilitation

Those setting up information systems for patients with spinal cord injury may find it valuable to draw from work developed by the National Spinal Cord Injury Statistical Center in Birmingham, Alabama, which is based on outcomes information from the model regional spinal cord injury care system program. A 20-year summary (1973–1992) of the uniform data set collected on new patients with spinal cord injury was published in late 1994 and includes data in the data base as of June 1, 1992. This material, organized according to the model spinal cord injury systems, includes annual follow-up data on 66,238 patients—estimated at 15% of all new SCI cases in the United States.[37]

As Doctor Stover noted in his 1993 Donald Munro Memorial Lecture of the American Paraplegia Society,[38] the demographics of spinal cord injury are gradually changing. While there may be some bias in the model system study because it is not a population-based study, these are the best prospective data now available in a large cohort of persons with spinal cord injury. In treating patients with spinal cord injury, one should obtain demographic, statistical, and outcome information that would dovetail with this study.

The annual incidence of spinal cord injury, not including those who die at the scene of the accident, is estimated to be between 30 and 40 cases per million population in the United States. Based on the 1992 census population of 254 million, these rates correspond to between 7600 and 10,000 new cases each year. The prevalence of spinal cord injury (the number of people in the United States alive today who have a spinal cord injury) has been estimated to be between 721 and 906 per million population. This corresponds to 183,000 to 203,000 persons.

The mean age of injury has increased from 28.5 years in 1973 to 33.4 years in 1992—an increase of 4.9 years (Fig. 7.7). The median age of the U.S. population has increased by an almost identical amount, meaning that persons injured are generally older, but there is no specific pattern of other change.

The greater than 4:1 ratio of male to female victims changed very little throughout the 20 years of model systems data collection. In 1973 the gender difference figures cited 81.9% men; there was an increase to 84.5% in the 1984 to 1986 period and, more recently, a decreased to 80.8%. Ethnic

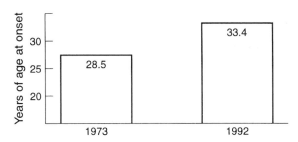

Figure 7.7. The mean age at initial spinal cord injury has increased by 4.9 years from 1973 to 1992.

group involvement has changed as well—possibly along with changes in diversity of the population as a whole. Between 1973 and 1977, 76.9% of persons in the database were Caucasian, 14% African American, 6.2% Hispanic, 2.1% American Indians, and 0.8% Asian American. Among those injured between 1990 and 1992, the proportion of Caucasians decreased to 56.3%, and the proportions of other ethnic groups increased: African American to 29.9%, Hispanics to 11.2%, and Asian Americans to 1.6%.

The etiology of spinal cord injury has changed with improvements in sports and vehicular safety as well as greater incidence of violence in our society. The percentage of such injuries due to motor vehicle crashes decreased from 47.2% in 1978–1980 to 38.1% in 1990–1992. The percentage of spinal cord injuries due to accidents during sporting events decreased from 14.8% to 8.8% in the same time frame. Showing a trend in the opposite direction, the percentage of spinal cord injuries due to acts of violence nearly doubled, from 13.9% to 25.1% (Fig. 7.8). Many feel that if the trend continues in this direction, violence will one day surpass vehicular accidents as the primary cause of spinal cord injury.

Violent acts more often cause paraplegia than quadriplegia. It is not clear whether this is why the percentage of cervical injuries decreased from 55.2% in 1981–1983 to 48.6% in 1990–1992 or whether other factors are responsible for this change. Paralleling advances in treatment, the percentage of complete spinal cord injuries declined from 55.7% in 1973–1977 to 45.7% in 1990–1992 (Fig. 7.9). This yields a greater potential for recovery of function. As testimony to improved care, the mortality rate declined by 42% over the last 20 years.

Improved delivery and efficiencies of care as well as advances in medicine have cut the length of initial hospital stay nearly in half, from 145 days in

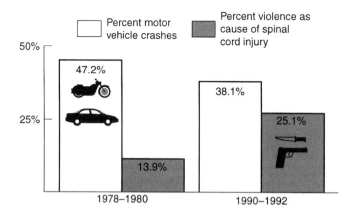

FIGURE 7.8. Acts of violence almost doubled as a cause of spinal cord injury and will one day be the primary cause if the trend continues.

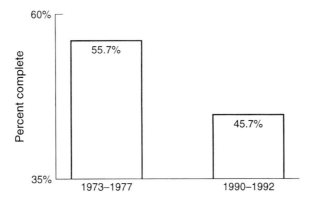

FIGURE 7.9. The 10% decline in complete spinal cord injuries from 1973 to 1992 yields a greater potential for recovery of function.

1973 to 77.5 days in 1992 (Fig. 7.10). However, inflation-adjusted costs of this care have raised hospital costs so that inflation-adjusted charges have increased despite a shorter length of stay. The initial hospital cost in 1973 (in 1992 dollars) was $91.947, and it had increased to $132,534 by 1990 (Fig. 7.11). Postdischarge care appears to be improving, as rehospitalization has declined from 11.7 days per year in 1973 to 4.4 days per year in 1989.

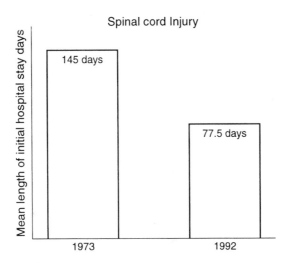

FIGURE 7.10. Initial hospital stay declined by 46.5% between 1973 and 1992.

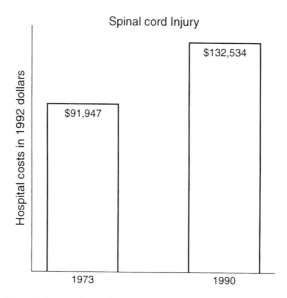

FIGURE 7.11. Hospital costs have increased despite shorter length of stay—yet not as fast as health care costs in general.

Life expectancy has dramatically improved. Before the early 1970s, renal failure was a primary cause of death for those with spinal cord injury, whereas now pulmonary complications—predominantly pneumonia and influenza—are the primary cause of death. These conditions account for 28.4% of deaths and are a second cause of death in an additional 3.5% of cases. The pathogenesis of pulmonary complications differs from other chronic lung conditions. Spinal cord–injured patients, hindered by weak exhalation, have difficulty expelling secretions. Patients with chronic lung disease, on the other hand, have primary difficulty in getting air and oxygen into the system. Pulmonary embolism is a subset of the pulmonary complications group and accounts for 8.3% of all deaths—predominantly during the first year after injury, whereas 3.8% of persons with spinal cord injury suffer a pulmonary embolism during the initial hospitalization. With earlier movement and intermittent catheterization and changes in treatment and equipment, complications such as penoscrotal abscesses and fistulas are almost nonexistent. Renal amyloidosis, felt to be a common cause of death 25 years ago, is now much less common.

It is noted that estimated costs depend on severity of injury and age and do not include any indirect costs, such as lost wages, fringe benefits, and productivity. The amount is felt to average almost $38,000, but it varies substantially based on education, severity of injury, and preinjury employment history.

TABLE 7.3. Life expectancy[a] for those who survive the first year postinjury, by severity of spinal cord injury and current age

Current age (years)	Normal	Tetraplegia		Paraplegia	Motor functional at any level
		High	Low		
20	56.3	32.8	38.6	44.8	49.0
30	46.9	26.8	30.7	36.7	40.5
40	37.6	20.9	23.6	28.8	31.7
50	38.6	15.5	17.0	21.2	23.4
60	20.5	11.0	11.2	13.8	15.9

[a]The life expectancy to the average remaining years of life for an individual. Among those with spinal cord injuries, life expectancies continue to increase, but are still somewhat below normal.

Life expectancy has increased, but is still somewhat below normal (Table 7.3). Moreover, mortality rates are significantly higher during the first year after injury than during subsequent years, particularly for severely injured persons.

Head Injury

Traumatic brain injury presents the greatest challenge to rehabilitation and to outcomes assessment because it is so variable. One cannot predict outcome with clinical exams and tests in TBI nearly as well as with spinal cord injury.

Mark Johnston and others discussed the use of various rating scales for evaluating traumatic brain injury.[39] The article covers measures of coma and global functioning [Glasgow Coma Scorle (GCS), Coma Recovery Scale (CRS), Rappaport Coma–Near Coma Scale, Western Neuro-Sensory Stimulation Profile (WNNS), Glasgow Outcome Scale (GOS), Rancho Los Amigos Level of Cognitive Function, Disability Rating Scale (DRS)] and disability measures, including the Functional Independence Measure (FIM), the Program Evaluation Conference System (PECS), the Barthel–Katz Index of Activities of Daily Living (ADL), the Community Living Assessment Scale (CLAS), the Lawton Instrumental Activities of Daily Living Scale, Older Americans Resources in Services (OARS), Bond's Social Scale, the Child Behavior Check List, the Vineland Adaptive Behavior Scale, the Neuro-Behavioral Rating Scale, the Frequency of Behaviors Scale, the Agitated Behavior Scale, and the Functional Assessment Inventory (FAI). Additionally, the article discusses measures of communication and cognitive function, and measures of handicap. Various types of validity, are covered, as well as the use of these tools in brain injury research and informatics models of outcomes measurement.

A study supported by the National Institute of Neurological Disorders and Stroke (NINDS) recognized that the Glasgow Outcome Scale for head injuries does not sufficiently distinguish among those who had received an outcome rating of "good."[40] The study, which looked at the variables that were most significantly correlated with success or failure in returning to school or work, effectively demonstrates the use of demographic and functional data to predict socially significant outcomes. (Incidentally, the three most potent predictors for return to work or school were intactness of the patient's verbal intellectual power, speed of information processing, and age.)

The disability rating scale developed by Rappaport et al.[41] in 1982 provides an evaluation system that measures function in the context of handicap. It is a continuous scale from 0 to 30 that can be effectively utilized as an outcome measurement in all head trauma patients. It is unfortunately limited to traumatic brain-injured patients, but provides a good standardized functional measure of these individuals. Interrater reliability is quite acceptable.

A study by Schalock and others looking at problems with information systems in state agencies dealing with brain-damaged clients is of interest.[42] Multiple problems were noted, including ineffective communication between user and developer, no systematic mechanism for translating policy questions to data-based form, inadequate systems due to ill-advised attempts to cut corners in the selection of hardware and software, problems with sharing database between systems, failures of different hardware systems to interact, poor reliability and validation in the system leading to inaccurate data, inadequate training, insufficient technical support, lack of user access, and overoptimistic projections of developmental time and cost. The article presents suggestions for dealing with these problems.

A national center for the study of traumatic brain injury was recently established at the University of Washington in Seattle. It is hoped that data on longitudinal head injury outcomes will one day be available and will be as useful as the data of the SCI model systems.

Specific Applications of Rehabilitation Informatics

Several studies have reviewed specific uses of informatics systems to facilitate intrahospital team communication or to simplify work for various therapies.

An interesting study from England describes an informatics system that allows the admissions office to enter demographic data initially, whereupon physicians and nurses enter history and signs and symptoms of handicapping conditions; laboratory and radiology staff enter relevant test results; and therapy services personnel enter function level and changes in outcome and response to treatment.[43]

The time spent in input is made up by eliminating the need for discharge summary by the various disciplines and the physician. Additionally, the system is reportedly quite easy to use.

It is felt to be a great help to have discharge summary available on the day of discharge with the push of a button. When this feature is available, relevant information can be quickly sent to home health services, housing authorities, social service departments, outpatient therapists, nursing homes, and all treating physicians.

Issues regarding confidentiality were discussed, including access to the system by patients and others who may want such information and the question of whether all medical information (e.g., positive tests for syphilis in a patient's distant past) had to be released with the comprehensive discharge summary.

The system is felt to be especially helpful for discharge planning by listing all issues that need to be addressed and requiring their completion before the report can be sent out. Follow-up functional status can be assessed by administering the "dependency questionnaire" to outpatients. The list of current medications, updated by Pharmacy, is included in the discharge summary.

One problem in rehabilitation is that the acuity needs for patients vary between and within diagnostic groups, resulting in the potential for great complexity. A. R. Gender, who describes the acuity system and classification tool developed by and for a nursing department of Sharp Memorial Hospital Rehabilitation Center in San Diego, California,[44] reports that the system has decreased staff nurses' time in rating patients, improved the accuracy of ratings, eased auditing, decreased clerical time, and improved management reports. Internal interrelater reliability has been facilitated, as well.

Parameters included ADLs/diet, mobility/activity, psychosocial parameters, treatments/procedures/equipment, medications and intravenous hookups, behavior/safety, psychosocial support, and bowel/bladder. Patients are given points based on the amount of care needed in each category, and these points are tabulated. Based on the number of points received, each patient is classified from 1 to 4, with 4 representing the highest level of nursing hours needed. The California users feel the tool has excellent ability to predict care needs for brain injury patients, but they observe that it congregates all quadriplegics at the high end of the level 4 range. Therefore, they recommend developing a fifth level to distinguish between quadriplegics to reflect the different care needs that are noted clinically.

Katherine McLaughlin and others prescribe an interesting approach to address self-care issues in a computerized nursing information system.[45] They that note the self-care deficit nursing theory presented by Orem[46] in 1985 readily lends itself to an informatics systems. This theory dovetails nicely with rehabilitation concepts, taking nursing from a medical model to a highly nursing-friendly model that addresses self-care skills and facilitates independence in a problem-oriented manner. This article and others following through it are highly recommended for those developing rehabilitative nursing informatics system.

Rudman and associates working in a group of Veterans Administration (VA) nursing homes developed a simple method to quantify changes in the ADLs over a 6-month time period in long-stay VA nursing home populations.[47] In this study, each resident was given a score based on the degree of independence in eating, mobility, transfers, and toileting. This "patient assessment instrument" (PAI) was scored from 1 to 5. Additionally, the program provides scores on bed sore status and on three types of abnormal behavior (inappropriate, verbally disruptive, and physically aggressive). Using this method, two nursing homes were compared as to whether residents improved, remained unchanged, or worsened.

A software program was developed that allowed the indicators from the PAI databank to automatically be input into the computer system of the information resource management service from the different VA medical centers. A report was generated every 6 months. Interestingly enough, the data showed that one of the nursing homes was much more successful than the other in maintaining functional levels. For further information on details of the system, contact Daniel Rudman (Department of Veterans Affairs, Clement J. Zablocki Medical College of Wisconsin, Medical and Information Resource Management Service, Milwaukee, WI 53295-1000.

Informatics can be helpful to physical therapists and other treating professionals who are "in the trenches" with patients and must make decisions about safety of therapy techniques. A medical history screening tool has been developed that helps the therapist recognize contraindications to specific therapy treatments.[48]

Farrell and Muik discuss the use of computers in the occupational therapy department to facilitate accumulation and analysis of patient information for test scoring, quality assurance, and management applications.[49] There is a detailed discussion of the computer as a tool to expedite the process of scoring a standardized test: the user first enters the numbers from the test tables into a Macintosh computer and then processes them by means of a spreadsheet program (Microsoft Excel, Version 3.0).

The test views include the developmental test of visual–motor integration (VMI), the Bruin Inks–Oseretsky Test of Motor Proficiency (BOTMP), the Peabody Developmental Motor Scale (PDMS), the Test of Visual Perceptual Skills (TVPS), and the Jebson Hand Function Test (JHFT). Additional uses of the tools discussed include using Microsoft Word to individualize home care instructions, tabulating and analyzing customer satisfaction by means of File Maker II, and using Claris HyperCard and File Maker II to categorize the department's software, videotape, and library collections.

An article by Soede discusses benefits of information technology to therapists in assessment and evaluation impairment, therapy training, and education.[50] For the disabled, information technology is felt to have tremendous future impact in allowing information access to and from remote databanks, facilitating direct person-to-person communications among patients with disabilities of speech and mobility, and facilitating the use of equipment such as manipulators, prosthetics, orthotics, mobility tools, and devices for the stimulation of paralyzed muscles. Going even beyond this area, Lim and others discussed the use of "virtual instruments" to test new therapy devices in the computer before they are even applied to patients.[51] Use of rehabilitative technologies in such advanced fields as visual perception, facilitation of human communication, prosthetics and orthotics, robotics, and signal processing was recently discussed.[52]

Environmental control systems and assistive devices based on microchip technology have been under development for the past two decades with excellent success.[14] Voice synthesizers have been developed to allow patients to communicate orally. Servo switches are operable by infrared telepathy to operate electronics devices such as light switches, televisions, automatic doors, and telephones. A recent development in this field has been the manufacture of a dental plate that is topped with a series of switches; this arrangement allows the person wearing the plate to operate a microcomputer-based environmental manipulation system by means of the tongue.[53]

Of course the advent of computers that respond to voice command alone opens up access to a wide variety of physically disabled people. Perhaps one of the more exciting recent developments in the field of rehabilitation informatics is the advent of imaging systems for the computer-aided design and manufacture of prosthetic devices for amputees.[54,55] These systems, which operate by x-ray, laser, or ultrasound, provide data acquisition and storage capability to the prosthetist in a competitively priced package for the provision of exact reproductions of a patient stump. This information enables the manufacture of the appropriate prosthesis in the shortest possible period of time.

Patient monitoring systems are most frequently used in intensive care units. In rehabilitation, there is work being done on systems to monitor patients for safety reasons. For example, patients who are confused and agitated may fall out of bed. There are infrared systems to detect movements and set off an alarm at the nursing station. This is an area of new development.

For the confused and agitated patient who is ambulatory and is at risk to walk off the unit, there are some systems that go beyond simple locked doors or alarms. A new monitor, worn on the patient's wrist, produces a readout on a computer system that permits a patient who wanders away from the unit to be located in or outside the hospital.

Monitoring systems for vital signs are not a major issue in the rehabilitation unit as they are in the intensive care unit.

Medical Record Systems

Medical records facilitate patient care by documenting history, observations, tests, plans, and procedures. They serve as a means of communication among attending physicians, consultants, nurses, and others. In the field of rehabilitation medicine, the chart is the primary focus for information shared by a multidisciplinary team of professionals. Different rehabilitation centers vary as to whether there are sections for the different therapies (physical therapy, occupational therapy, speech pathology, psychology, social services, cognitive rehabilitation, neuropsychology, recreational therapy, behavioral medicine, rehabilitation counseling, vocational evaluation, driver's evaluation, work hardening, respiratory therapy, and rehabilitation nursing), or whether all therapy notes are compiled in chronological order in one section. Usually there is a section for the interdisciplinary team conference. This material includes the initial evaluations when goals are established, interim conferences, and final or discharge conferences. There may be conferences with or without the physician, and with or without the patient and family members. Trauma centers and rehabilitation centers vary greatly with respect to membership of the rehabilitation team and the nature of team conferences.

While computerized medical records have not supplanted the regular charts in most rehabilitation hospitals, use of computers to supplement certain departmental operations is rapidly growing. For example, systems exist to facilitate the reporting of the multidisciplinary team conferences. Goals of various disciplines are brought into a unified treatment plan and are kept in a computer. These main problem areas, with treatment goals, are then reviewed weekly with updated notes on progress toward achievement of the goals. This type of reporting turns a multidisciplinary team into what on paper appears to be an interdisciplinary team—the entire team working together toward common goals.

In other settings, various therapies may enter their initial reports on a computer. This material can be used to expedite the writing of the discharge summary. Computers can be used to document daily progress notes and to record the patient contact hours. Some hospitals are working to help the therapist save time by compiling these daily notes into a weekly team conference report. Programs now exist to use the entered data on patient charges and contact hours to generate a management report indicating the number of total contact hours generated by an individual therapist. This breakdown is useful in determining the efficiency of therapists' use of a most valuable resource—their time. Such data can be used in productivity analyses as well as to determine the need for hiring additional therapists.[56]

While the capability is not readily available, many rehabilitation centers hope to be able to have data analyzed such that therapists can have their own FIM scores tabulated for purposes of determining individual efficacy in the treatment. When one works often with therapists, one realizes that some are much more effective than others in working with the physical and emotional aspects of their patients to help them achieve as much independence as possible within the limitations of their disabilities. Therapy is still much an art, and thus a management tool such as this is helpful for administrators as well as rehabilitation physicians to determine whether they have the right staffing to optimize rehabilitation outcomes.

The computer-stored medical record has potential advantages in accessibility. Specifically, records generated by one department can be accessed by another. A physician with an office terminal who must discuss a patient's rehabilitative progress with an insurance company official for the purpose of determining the need for continued stay can review the most up-to-date records without running back to the hospital or calling each therapy department. Likewise, the rehabilitation hospital case manager or social worker can have access to updated progress toward goals in reporting to fellow insurance nurses. Computerized charting has facilitated the tedious daily documentation required of rehabilitation nurses, who are responsible for the day-to-day carryover of rehabilitation skills learned in therapy to the "real world" of the nursing floor. For example, a patient who has a head injury and inattention to the left side may be working on left-hemisphere inattention. When this patient is eating in the dining room, the clever nurse puts the dessert on the left side.

Nursing is also responsible for monitoring safety and ensuring that transfer skills are reinforced. Nursing must also monitor bowel and bladder function and work on these to optimize independence. Rather than manually rewriting goals and functions every day, there areas can be included in the daily printout of the care plan, with updates made where progress has occurred. Computer-based systems such as this provide better organized and more legible reports. The software imposes structure on the data and, through a system of asking questions and leaving blanks to be filled in, ensures that data are more complete. This feature may be helpful in the medical–legal realm as well, by ensuring that all relevant questions are asked. Some computer systems can essentially "refuse" to go on the next screen until all relevant information has been provided.

For centers that are using clinical/critical pathways, the computer can assure that all relevant information is entered. This form of backup is also important for the collection of FIM data, since an evaluative tool that misses even one element is invalid and not eligible to be entered into the system. An interactive system could even help a center go beyond the limitations of management tools by prompting the use of additional information. For example, in classifying spinal cord–injured patients, the FIMS lumps C-5 through C-8 quadriplegics. As everyone in rehabilitation knows, these levels vary dramatically and have substantial differences in expected outcomes (i.e., C-5 is not a C-6 is not a C-7 is not a C-8). An ideal system could prompt the user to enter the patient's exact neurologic level, and thus outcomes data could be better compared to expected outcomes for spinal cord injury at the level indicated.

Interactive computer systems are used in at least one center to generate reports of modified swallowing studies for dysphagia. The computer asks a series of questions, and the speech pathologist fills in the answers. The computer then uses the data to generate a report in narrative form. The report has the advantage of having a consistent style and being thorough. If one initially generates a clear and cohesive report with no spelling errors, it will always come out as a clear, cohesive report with no spelling errors—the opposite is also true!

Additionally, information that is generated in reports of this type can be easily aggregated for the purposes of outcomes measurement and clinical research.

A medical record system that uses computers has the disadvantages of a large initial investment to cover the computer hardware, software, and training costs. Most rehabilitation centers find the need to customize the new system in some way to meet their particular needs. However, having information stored in computer memory rather than in one medical file is a threat to confidentiality because the material is accessible to anyone with a terminal or modem. Thus users must have a means to ensure confidentiality through the use of passwords, code words, and other such methods. Of course with computers there is potential for delays with "downtime", so it is helpful to have backup paper records. Yet another barrier to the widespread use of computerized medical records systems is the potential for error inherent in manual data entry. This can be eliminated if data can be directly captured from the source in machine-readable form. To take advantage of this advance in technology, forms must be standardized and made user-friendly, as well as digitally efficient.

A computer software package called Teleform exists for business applications to create and fax forms. At the University of Tennessee Medical Center at Knoxville, a nurse named Thomas Hutzenbiler used this system in the development of clinical pathways.[57] Physician input was obtained to develop clinical pathway recommendations, and this work led to standardized admission orders for certain diagnoses. This in turn generated nursing orders and progress notes. Information generated from physician selection of orders and choices in nursing progress notes is then collected and summarized on a machine-readable quality assurance form. If the computer cannot identify a particular handwritten entry, it flags Mr. Hutzenbiler, who then scans the form to decipher the imperfect penmanship. This leads directly into quality assurance data and a means to monitor the implementation of clinical pathways.

There are a variety of means to prevent errors.[58] One is to program the system to scrupulously apply validity checks. *Range checks* can detect or prevent entry values that are out of range (e.g., a serum-potassium level of 50.0). Pattern checks can verify that the entered data have the required pattern (e.g., the three digits followed by a hyphen and then four digits of a local telephone number). *Computed checks* can verify that values have the correct mathematical relationship; thus white blood cell differential counts (reported as percentages) must sum to 100. *Consistency checks* can compare entered data to detect errors (e.g., the recording of impotence as a diagnosis for a spinal cord–injured woman). *Delta checks* warn of large and unlikely differences between the value of a new result and the preceding observation (e.g., a recorded weight that changes by 100lb in 2 weeks). Better known are *spelling checks*, which verify the spelling of individual words.[58]

There has been much resistance to the use of automated medical record systems. They are cumbersome in data entry and expensive in start-up costs. However, as health care systems aggregate into larger groups (managed care situations, health maintenance organizations, etc.), the larger institutions will tend to invest in these systems to benefit from economies of scale and centralized management of clinical and administrative data.

One area of resistance entails the entry of physician-collected data into the system. There are three current methods:

1. Transcription of physicians' notes (especially pertinent when the practice has already invested in dictation services) is particularly helpful if physicians follow a standard form in which a transcriptionist can enter dictated reports into a modestly structured computer record.[58]

2. Use by physicians of a structured encounter form from which their notes are transcribed (possibly coded) by support personnel. To date, this has reportedly been the most successful approach.

3. Direct entry of data by a physician working at a video display terminal. This has been best accepted by physicians (e.g., surgeons in the postoperative setting), who can enter standard orders to cover the requirements of most patients. Where greater time is required to enter data than would be required to write the same information manually, physicians have been reluctant to use the computer systems.

The lengthy process of entering patient histories, physical findings, and progress notes has stood as a major obstacle to acceptance of computer-based medical records by physicians, who are reasonably jealous of their limited time.

McDonald and Barnett see the day when the physicians working at a microcomputer-based medical workstation linked to a hospital can gather medical information, lists of medications, lab test results, information on drug interactions, the latest articles relevant to that diagnosis, and databases of expert opinions. They visualize physicians of the future being able to "find all the information they need linked in one seamless web, available at any time through their medical-record work stations."[58]

Until quite recently, hospital information systems have remained mostly at the level of support services such as billing, patient registration, and tracking inventory and staffing, as well as getting information from the laboratory and radiology departments to the floors. Newly evolving hospital information systems are promising to facilitate data entry by physicians as well as supporting clinical research. Point-of-care systems provide bedside terminals that allow nurses and physicians to record data as they collect information from the patient. Potentially, these systems could increase the productivity of nurses by reducing the amount of paperwork and providing more accurate and timely access to detailed clinical information for quality assurance activities. This capability is just beginning to be used by a few rehabilitation hospitals.

Biographic Retrieval Systems

Biographic retrieval systems are an important area of informatics. One cannot read, memorize, and recall all information necessary for high quality medical practice—let alone for research. The literature has grown exponentially: in the biomedicine area, there are more than 20,000 journals and 17,000 new books published annually.

Computer technology is increasingly being used to facilitate rapid and convenient access to the literature. MEDLINE is the National Library of Medicine's major bibliographic database. This computer-based system contains more than 900,000 references to recent literature. Its files, dating back to 1966, contain more than 6 million citations and are available for searches. More than 4 million searches are conducted annually.

The National Library of Medicine references 3400 medical journals with over 340,000 articles annually. On-line searching is faster and more cost efficient than retrieving these references through the printed Index Medicus. With on-line searching, one can locate articles dealing with two or more topics at a time—a mode of retrieval that would be vary tedious with Index Medicus. The National Library of Medicine divides the country into seven regions, each served by a regional medical library. One uses the MEDLINE by consulting a reference book entitled "Medical Subject Headings" (MeSH), which lists the categorized headings and subheadings as well as cross-references. One then uses these key terms to locate various references. The MEDLARS (Medical Literature Analysis and Retrieval System) Medicine project of the National Library of offers an annotated list of over 315,000 articles per year covering 2800 journals.

Other biomedical databases, listed by Siegel et al.[59] include:

1. Biosis Previews, produced by Bioscience Information Service. Abstracts from 1969 to the present covering worldwide literature and research in the life sciences.
2. EMBASE, the on-line database of Excerpta Medica, has operated since 1974—now abstracting over 3.5 million records and covering about 4500 journals.

3. Psychinfo has from 1967 through the present covered over 1500 books, 950 journals, and other materials from the world's literature on psychology and the behavioral sciences. It is produced by the American Psychological Association.

Grateful Med is a microcomputer software package in a user-friendly format allows access to MEDLINE and CATLINE (catalog records for books and journals), AVLINE (audiovisual materials for health education), AIDSLINE, DIRALINE (a directory of organizations that provide information for the general public), and a variety of other National Library of Medicine databases. Grateful Med is an easy-to-use and relatively inexpensive approach to computer searches.[59,60]

A recent study looked at which information service was the most comprehensive in recognizing articles in the rehabilitation literature.[61] The British Library's Current Awareness Topic Service (CATS) was felt to be the most comprehensive. Others studied included MEDLINE, Excerpta Medica, Cinahal (Cumulative Insights to Nursing and Allied Health), Serline (Serials Online, National Library of Medicine), Sachet (British Library Serials Database), and Ulrich's International Periodicals Directory. The number of core journals in rehabilitation is very large, and their coverage by information services is very selective Altogether, a total of 111 different journals were found that deal with rehabilitation topics. However, even this study grossly underestimated rehabilitative coverages that included no non–English language journals.

Davis and Findley[62] present a nice discussion about the use of different databases to access the rehabilitative literature with topics including amputee rehabilitation, spinal cord injury rehabilitation, traumatic brain injury rehabilitation, decubitus care, rehabilitation engineering, pain rehabilitation, and sexual rehabilitation, using the Grateful Med Software for Simplified Online Medline Searches. Also discussed are Excerpta Medica, Scisearch (Science Citation Index), ABLEDATA, Hyper ABLEDATA (for use with the Macintosh HyperCard system), Psychological Abstracts, Conference Papers Index, CRISP, ERIC, Rehab Data, Sport Database, Engineering Index, VA Rehabilitation R&D Database, Ageline (covering social gerontology, a combined health information database), linguistics and language behavior abstracts, OT Source, and the United Nations Disability Statistics Database (covering 95 countries). A number of foreign language journals are also reviewed in this article.

The growth of medical literature has made direct access to computerized searches more important. Systems have developed to allow individual physicians and other professionals to access these databases directly rather than going through professional librarians or other professionals and library staff. This improvement has been facilitated by the development of user-friendly software that is menu driven—that is, not requiring memorization of large amounts of off-screen data. For more information in this area, see the text on end user searches edited by Wood et al.[63] Some helpful sources include Mini Medline[64] and Paperchase.[65] There is also the Epilepsy Abstracts Retrieval System (EARS) available for those interested in seizure disorders—head injury being the most common cause of seizures.

For those interested in acquiring access to a bibliographic retrieval service, Sewell* points out that to allow physicians, paraprofessionals, and other "end users" to directly access search services, it is to necessary expand three factors:

1. *Awareness.* Potential users should know what is out there and what they would be missing if an "overly simplistic system" were chosen.

2. *Accessibility to the work site.* Sometimes subsets of MEDLINE are available locally. Sewell recommends that vendors "provide immediate and direct access to the full text of the paper once a reference to it has been found. Other display capabilities should be more flexible than they are at present."

3. *Assistance.* The librarian should be familiar with the hardware and software used, as well as health science databases, which should be readily available for help in end user searching.

How does one properly search a rehab topic? The subheadings from MeSH can be "exploded," or expanded, to find related topics. "Explosions," Sewell notes, "increase recall by collecting hierarchically subsidiary terms when a single term is exploded." On the other hand, "Subheadings improve precision by subdividing the topic of a term into just one aspect of it." Failure to properly explode topics accounts for errors in over half of searches and causes searchers to find less than a third of what they would have liked to retrieve. The same Maryland study of health professionals' difficulties with MEDLINE searches indicates that users had problems with finding proper subheadings only 13% of the time. Searchers who encounter such difficulties, however, miss 85% or more of the data they are searching.

Writing specifically on rehabilitation, Bohannon[67] notes that "many topics do not have specific medical subject headings that relate to them (e.g., muscle strength) . . . [and] finding an article through the use of the medical subject headings of index medicus may be cumbersome, time consuming, and difficult." He recommends use of the Permuterm Index of Scientific Citation Index to locate articles, since titles include specific topical words or phrases. Another source to follow up on articles written by specific authors is the Sources Index of Science Citation Index. To find other articles that your author of index cites, use the Citation Index of Science Citation Index.

---

*In Reference 66, which is the source of all quotations from Sewell in this section.

There is now an electronic bulletin board that focuses on general information and referral for the disabled. It addresses a variety of issues, including equipment exchange, legislation, medical information, nutrition, self-help, and specialty services. Public message access permits participants to interact. Called Alliance, the service can be connected by contacting Rick Dayton, 38 North Oakdale, #12, Medford, Oregon 27501, or calling (503) 779-4158.[68]

One can access the National Rehabilitation Information Center (NARIC), the publisher of ABLEDATA, a computerized listing of commercially available devices for rehabilitation and independent living, by calling 1-800-34-NARIC or writing NARIC, 4407 Eighth Street, NE, Washington, DC 20017.

An interactive videodisk catalogue of products and services for persons with disabilities, ProDisc Acero, is reached by fax at (404) 874-8433 or by calling (404) 872-9700.

Limitations of the Classification Systems and Needs for the Future

For data to be useful, diagnoses must be well defined as well as uniformly applied and accepted. The federal Health Care Financing Administration publishes a national diagnostic coding scheme, the current version of which is the Ninth International Classification of Disease (ICD-9, 1990). All non-military hospitals in the United States must use these codes for discharge coding purposes. The ICD-9 codes do not come close to defining cases sufficiently to lump them for study purposes and rehabilitation. Functional Independence Measure Scales (FIMS) make some attempt to do this, but the system falls short.

For example, as noted earlier, the system for coding spinal cord injuries does not sufficiently distinguish between the different levels of spinal cord function. All quadriplegics are lumped into two groups: C-1 to C-4 and C-5 to C-8. In real life, patients with complete C-3 quadriplegia or higher are ventilator-dependent, while those with C-4 are able to leave ventilator support but have no arm function. C-5 quadriplegics have elbow function and can use universal cuffs for ADLs, but require help for physical needs such as transfers and bladder and bowel care. Patients with C-6 level function can do most of their activities of daily living and use writing utensils quite adroitly with training. Some at this level can be independent in most transfer skills and even do intermittent catheterization. A few can live alone. Many require help. C-7 quadriplegics who are in good physical condition can often be independent in transfers and self-care skills and therefore are able live alone. Yet they have limitations in respiratory function. Patients with C-8 quadriplegia are the first level to begin to have some good intrinsic hand function. Additionally, some patients have one level on one side and a different level on the other; others have an incomplete type of quadriplegia such as a central cord syndrome, the Brown–Séquard syndrome, superimposed on their basic level of quadriplegia. Superimposed conditions such as elbow fractures that limit extension or heterotopic ossification can modify the functional potential. These factors are not sufficiently considered in any system used for coding.

Like many other professional organizations focusing on a particular condition, the American Spinal Injury Association (ASIA) has developed a classification system that appropriately separates the types of spinal cord injury. Perhaps this level of sophistication is needed to analyze patients appropriately to predict functional outcomes. So many different levels of classification are required, however, that those not intimately familiar with the system may find it cumbersome. Such terms as "ASIA motor score" (which gives a numerical rank to the spinal cord injury level) are completely foreign to practitioners outside the area of spinal cord injury care. Applying such a complicated system to trauma centers and later attempting to carry it over to rehabilitation centers almost surely would be futile. For most trauma centers, it is infrequent to find the spinal cord injury levels consistently and accurately classified.

By analogy, pathologists have developed their own widely used coding system—SNOMED, the Systematized Nomenclature of Medicine. So detailed that it provides more than 50 separate codes for describing tuberculosis infections, SNOMED permits coding of pathological findings in exquisite detail. It contains no codes for radiologic findings such as the details of an x-ray film of the colon, however. Therefore,

In a particular clinical setting, not one of the common coding schemes is likely to be completely satisfactory. In some cases, the granularity of the code will be too coarse. . . . On the other hand, another practitioner may prefer to aggregate many individual codes . . . into a single category to simplify the coding and retrieval of data.

Such schemes cannot be effective unless they are accepted by health care providers. There is an inherent tension between the need for a coding system that is general enough to cover many individual patients and the need for precise and unique terms that accurately apply to a specific patient and do not unduly constrain physicians' attempts to describe what they observe.[69]

Yet if a physician's view of the computer-based medical record is a blank sheet of paper on which any unstructured information can be written, the data of the record will be unsuitable for dynamic processing, clinical research, and health planning. The challenge is to learn how to meet all these needs through a common structure that ties together the various vocabularies that have been created. Researchers at many institutions are currently working to develop such a unified medical language system. It is unlikely, however, that any such system will be readily applicable to the diagnosis of disability in the field of rehabilitation medicine in the near future. Those looking at outcome data may not realize the profound impact of social factors on disability if such parameters as return to work are considered. Persons with mild memory or attention deficits may be able to return to employment as laborers without great difficulties, yet in such fields as engineering and journalism, where new information must be consistently and rapidly processed, the same deficits would be incapacitating.

Anyone who works extensively with different tools to measure functional outcomes and program evaluations is impressed with the trade-off among systems. Systems that best look at function are those aimed at a specific diagnosis. Once a system has been expanded to look at several diagnoses, sensitivity is often lost. Can one truly compare the level of improvement in function in a head-injured person who goes from coma to walking and talking to the kinds of improvement on the same scale for a spinal cord–injured patient at the C-5 level who starts and leaves dependent in transfers and in whom the major goals might be ADL improvements involving the hands with adaptations? Primary rehabilitation issues in someone with quadriplegia at this level revolve around educating the patient and caregiver regarding aspects of care—in bowel, bladder, and pulmonary functions, and in nutrition. A scale sensitive enough to show changes in one diagnosis may overly minimize changes with another diagnosis.

Using a highly expanded measurement system to classify injuries to the head and spinal cord is analogous to trying to measure all distances with a ruler. Imagine distances between stars and distances between atomic particles all in feet—the numbers would be ridiculous. To some extent the problem is even worse with patients of certain types, as one discovers when, say, measuring levels of improvement in head-injured patients at Rancho Los Amigos Level IV (confused and agitated) or measuring the improvements in acceptance and knowledge of the condition for those with spinal cord injury. These situations do not lend themselves to traditional measuring tools at all. To insist on applying them is like trying to describe musical notes with a ruler. It just does not make sense. Yet these are the data we submit to third-party payers and reviewers and ask them to make decisions about appropriateness of rehabilitation. The ideal system will have a measurement tool appropriate to the diagnosis and compare patients with similar diagnoses. This has not been achieved in the twentieth century.

The currently available systems for classifying severity of injury fails to take into account issues that have a substantial impact in functional outcome. Rather, they consider medical conditions resulting in death or morbidity in a more general sense, such as a prolonged hospital stay. An optimal measuring system that included rehabilitation issues would take into account the specific presenting condition and its likely possible outcomes. In certain conditions—particularly neurological injury or loss of a limb—certain outcomes and limitations are predictable results of a given injury. Basically, when Humpty Dumpty falls off the wall, it does not matter who are the doctors, nurses, horses, or men who attempt to put the pieces together, one can only go so far.

Recognizing these limitations, one can use currently available tools to measure functional outcomes. Rehabilitation has been at the forefront of medical sciences in dealing with functional outcomes. Other disciplines also addressing these issues include oncology, which has developed the Karnofsky Scale to measure level of function versus needs for assistance and care. However, even this scale may not distinguish between a head-injured person who is so disabled he is able only to eat and do little else and a middle-aged C-6 quadriplegic who needs help with bowel, bladder, and transfers but can drive a van to work every day and help raise a family and pay taxes.

The developments discussed in this chapter will serve to open the door to further research and development in the field of rehabilitation informatics. In the near future, physiatrists will be able to plan rehabilitation programs with more efficiency and more success than ever before. Additional information will be available for the determination of the most effective and efficient utilization of resources, and the trauma victim will be returned to the highest level of function in the shortest period of time.

Appendix

Medical Record Systems

There are various automated ambulatory medical record systems in existence.[69] COSTAR, developed by Barnett and colleagues at the Massachusetts General Hospital to support the Harvard Community Health Plan, has been used in more than 110 separate installations. In 1978, after revisions for use by other ambulatory care practices, it was made available to any organization that wanted to use or market the product. There is a public domain version, as well as many enhanced commercial versions. COSTAR includes modules for system security and data integrity, patient registration, appointment scheduling, billing and financial reporting, collection and storage of medical records, management reporting, and pharmacy. Prior to a scheduled patient visit, the system prints out a summary medical record for review by the physician as well as a blank encounter form to be used to capture administrative and medical data from the visit. After a visit, clerical personnel enter the data from the form onto the computer system.

The Regenstreif Medical Record System (RMRS), developed by McDonald and colleagues at Indiana University Medical Center, has been used since 1974. A unique feature is a reminder system that reviews patient data and produces reminder notes for the physician based on 1400 definitions and coded protocol rules. The system prompts physicians to order laboratory tests when appropriate and to prescribe or modify medication plans. It produces three documents prior to the patient's visit:

1. A quality assurance report, which contains recommendations to the physician about preventive procedures that should be performed and the problems to be evaluated.
2. A flowsheet summary—a time-ordered summary of the clinical database.
3. The patient encounter form, to capture new medical data during the visit. Also included are active prescriptions and commonly ordered tests.

A data entry clerk is needed to record the flowsheet observations into the clinical database. Another alternative is to just save the paper record.

The Medical Record (TMR), developed by Stead and Hammond at Duke University in 1975, provides appointment-scheduling and billing capabilities. It is used at over 25 sites in the United States and Canada. TMR is similar to other systems except that physicians are encouraged to enter their prescriptions directly into the record—thus taking advantage of the system's ability to warn against drug allergies and interactions and to calculate correct dosages. TMR can display data in one of three ways: problem, time, or encounter. Doctors can view sequential values of a finding or test.

The Summary Time Oriented Record (STOR) was developed by Whiting–O'Keefe and Associates at the University of California at San Francisco. STOR supports 22 clinic locations with 200,000 outpatient visits per year. The system displays computer-based storage and retrieval of ambulatory medical records and on-line display of inpatient and outpatient clinical information and response to user queries. Before each clinic visit, STOR updates its database and prints a patient-specific encounter form. If clinic-defined criteria are met (about 25% of visits), STOR orders retrieval of the paper medical record.

The University of Utah has developed the HELP system to meet clinical teaching and research needs of hospital personnel. Warner and colleagues developed it for use at the teaching hospital in Latter Day Saints Hospital, a teaching hospital in Salt Lake City, Utah (see Fig. 7.12).*

HELP provides decision support in the form of knowledge frames, which are specialized decision logic modules that permit the computer to react to data as they are entered in a patient's files, and thus to generate patient-specific warnings, alerts, diagnostic suggestions, and limited management advice. HELP protocols also can be written to evaluate the patient's database and set periodic intervals (e.g., to check whether a patient who is

---

*For a discussion of HELP, and for the source of all this sections quotations about the PROMIS system, see Reference 69.

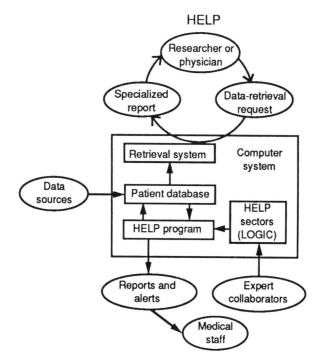

FIGURE 7.12. In HELP, the typical functions of a hospital information system are augmented by HELP frames that encode decision logic. When data in the patient database satisfy the preconditions of a frame, the program generates an advisory report or warning. (From Shortliffe EH, Perreault LE, eds. *Medical Informatics: Computer Applications in Health Care.* Reading, MA: Addison-Wesley; 1990:236.)

receiving a potassium-wasting diuretic has had his serum-potassium level measured during a prespecified time).

The Problem-Oriented Medical Information System (PROMIS: Fig. 7.13) was developed by Weed and colleagues at the University of Vermont.

PROMIS was designed to be used routinely by physicians in lieu of all paper record keeping. Physicians used a computer terminal not only to order tests and drugs but also to record and review medical histories, data collected during physical examinations, progress notes and the like. PROMIS actively guided the interaction taking steps to insure that the data entered were complete, were entered according to conventions that would allow the physician's logic to be apparent ... (PROMIS) was designed to replace all paper records and to enhance uniformity and quality of care.

PROMIS implemented Weed's vision of the problem solving medical record, record in which all diagnostic and therapeutic actions are tied to underlying patient problem. This philosophy was expressed in a collection of strictly defined logic pathways for data collection problem solving. At each point in a computer session, a user was presented with a set of related choices. When the user selected an item, the information was recorded in the medical records; the program's logic that determine which screen of related choices was presented next.

Of the three systems [HELP, PROMIS, and COSTAR], PROMIS clearly had the most sophisticated user interface and the greatest capacity to structure and organize medical information. Yet, in part because of the dogmatic and inflexible nature of the system, PROMIS was not well accepted by its physician users and is not used in any major hospital today.

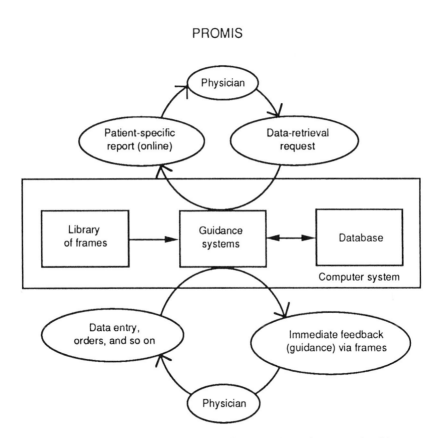

FIGURE 7.13. All interaction with PROMIS occurs through a central guidance system. The system updates and retrieves patient information from the database using a special library of *frames* that encode the guidance logic. Each frame fills one computer terminal screen; the physician can select options by touching the touch-screen display. The order of frames to be displayed is determined by the options that the physician has selected on earlier screens. Both data retrieval and data entry follow this same interactive scheme. (From Shortliffe EH, Perreault LE, eds. *Medical Informatics: Computer Applications in Health Care.* Reading, MA: Addison-Wesley; 1990:238.)

The lessons of the PROMIS system are that too great a structure in physician interaction breaks down as a result of the complexity of individual patient needs. The system needs to be flexible enough to allow the physician to make appropriate decisions in response to the real clinical picture and the complexities of real people with more than one presenting condition, as well as the complexities of the social–psychological milieu. In fact, this has been the problem with hospital information systems as a whole: There is "a poor fit between problem and solution (that) causes poor user acceptance of the system."[69] Nevertheless, in 1985 over 200 vendors were supplying information systems or services to hospitals.

Clinical and administrative demands in combination with increasing capabilities with advancements in technology will result in the development of sophisticated information systems. Cost containment is a double-edged sword—hospitals feel the need to have good information, but they worry about major expenditures in this area. In short, there may be less and less ability to tolerate errors in system selection. As Friedman and Martin point out, "There is a need for physicians to actively participate in strategic policy making and selection and development of relevant hospital information systems."[70]

Additional information on COSTAR or PROMIS may be obtained by writing to Policy Implications of Medical Informatics Systems, Government Printing Office, U.S. Office of Technology, Washington, D.C. 20401.

Acknowledgment. The authors express their appreciation also to Samuel R. Stover, MD, professor and Chairman of Rehabilitation Medicine, University of Alabama at Birmingham, and director of the National SCI Statistical Center, Birmingham, Alabama.

References

1. Rusk HA. Rehabilitation. *JAMA* 1949;140:287–292.
2. Granger CV. Health accounting—Functional assessment of the long-term patient. In: Kottke FJ, Stillwell GK, Lehmann JF, eds. *Krusen's Handbook of Physical Medicine and Rehabilitation*, 3rd ed. Philadelphia: WB Saunders; 1982:253.
3. Mahoney FI, Barthel DW. Functional evaluation: Barthel Index. *Maryland State Med J* 1965;14:61–65.
4. Katz S, Downs TD, Cash HR, et al. Progress in development of index of ADL. *Gerontologist* 1970;10:20–30.
5. Schoening HA, Iversen IA. Numerical scoring of self-care status: A study of Kenny Self-Care Evaluation. *Arch Phys Med Rehabil* 1968;49:221–229.
6. Moskowitz E, McCann CB. Classification of disability in the chronically ill and aging. *J Chronic Dis* 1957;5:324–346.
7. Granger CV, Greer DS. Functional status measurements in medical rehabilitation outcomes. *Arch Phys Med Rehabil* 1976;57:103–109.

8. Fortinsky RH, Granger CV, Seltzer GB. The use of functional assessment in understanding home care needs. *Med Care* 1981;19:489–497.
9. Harvey RF, Jellinek HM. Functional performance assessment: A program approach. *Arch Phys Med Rehabil* 1981;62:456–461.
10. Jond G, Hughes J. Independent living: Methodology for measuring long-term outcomes. *Arch Phys Med Rehabil* 1982;63:68–73.
11. Granger CV, Albrecht GL, Hamilton BB. Outcome of comprehensive medical rehabilitation: Measurement by PULSES Profile and the Barthel Index. *Arch Phys Med Rehabil* 1979;60:145–154.
12. Commission on Accreditation of Rehabilitation Facilities. *Standards Manuals.* Tucson, AZ: CARF; 1992:7–8; 1994:14–16, 18–20, 57–70.
13. Williamson JW. *Assessing and Improving Health Care Outcomes: The Health Accounting Approach to Quality Assurance.* Cambridge, MA: Ballinger; 1978.
14. DeLisa J, ed. *Rehabilitation Medicine: Principles and Practice*, 2nd ed. Philadelphia: JB Lippincott; 1993.
15. Gill TM, Feinstein AR. A critical appraisal of the quality of quality-of-life measurements. *JAMA* 1994;272(8):619–626.
16. World Health Organization. *International Classification of Impairments, Disabilities, and Handicaps: A Manual of Classification Relation to the Consequences of Disease.* Geneva: WHO; 1980.
17. American Medical Association. *Guides to the Evaluation of Permanent Impairment*, 4th ed. Chicago: AMA; 1993.
18. Pope AM, Tarlov AR, eds. *Disability in America: Toward a National Agenda for Prevention.* Washington, DC: National Academy Press; 1991.
19. Pope AM, Tarlof AR, eds. *Disability in America: Toward a National Agenda for Prevention.* Washington, DC: National Academy Press; 1991:165.
20. Audet AM, Scott HD. The Uniform Clinical Data Set: An evaluation of the proposed national database for medicine's quality review program. *Ann Intern Med* 1993;119:1209–1213.
21. Johnson MV, Keith RA, Hinderer SR. Measurement standards for interdisciplinary medical rehabilitation. *Arch Phys Med Rehabil* 1992;73:S1–S21.
22. Granger CV, Gresham GE. New developments in functional assessment. *PMR Clin North Am* August 1993.
23. Granger CV, Hamilton BB, Sherwin FS. *Guide for Use of the Uniform Data Set for Medical Rehabilitation.* Buffalo, NY: Uniform Data System for Medical Rehabilitation; 1986.
24. Hamilton BB, Granger CV, Sherwin FS, Sielenzny M, Tashman MJ. A Uniform National Data System for Medical Rehabilitation. In: Fuhrer MJ, ed. *Rehabilitation Outcomes: Analysis and Measurement.* Baltimore: Paul H Brookes; 1987:137–147.
25. Granger CV, Hayes M, Johnson M, Deutsch A, Braun S, Fiedler RC. Quality and outcome measures for medical rehabilitation. In: Bradden R, Buschbacher R, eds. *Krusen's Handbook of Physical Medicine and Rehabilitation*, 3rd ed. Philadelphia: WB Saunders; 1997.
26. Granger CV, Hamilton BD. The Uniform Data System for Medical Rehabilitation Report of First Admissions for 1992. *Am J Phys Med Rehabil* 1994;73:51–55.

27. Granger CV. Personal communication, 1994.
28. Kaiser LR. Key management skills for the physician executive. In: Curry W, ed. *The Physician Executive*. Tampa, FL: American College of Physician Executives; 1988:78–101.
29. Klint RB, Long HW. Costs/quality relationships: A generic model for health care. In: Curry W, ed. *The Physician Executive*. Tampa, FL: American College of Physician Executives; 1988:159–175.
30. Rodriguez AR. Maintaining quality in the cost-conscious environment. In: Curry W, ed. *The Physician Executive*. Tampa, FL: American College of Physician Executives; 1988:191–206.
31. Iezzoni LI. Severity standardization and hospital quality assessment. In: Couch JB, ed. *Health Care Quality Management for the Twenty-First Century*. Tampa, FL: American College of Physician Executives; 1991:177–234.
32. Joint Commission for the Accreditation of Healthcare Organizations. *Accreditation Manual for Hospitals*. Chicago: JCAHO; 1994.
33. Lipson EH. Guidelines for medical quality management program development. In: Couch JB, ed. *Physician Managers and the Law: Legal Aspects of Medical Quality Management*. Tampa, FL: American College of Physician Executives; 1989.
34. Couch JB, Rodriguez AR. Legal aspects of clinical outcome management. In: Couch JB, ed. *Physician Managers and the Law: Legal Aspects of Medical Quality Management*. Tampa, FL: American College of Physician Executives; 1989:38–47.
35. Shortliffe EH, Barnette GO. Medical data: Their acquisition, storage and use. In: Shortliffe EH, Perreault LE, eds. *Medical Informatics: Computer Applications in Health Care*. Reading, MA: Addison-Wesley; 1990:55.
36. Pine M. The use of large databases to monitor and manage the quality of health care. In: Couch JB, ed. *Health Care Quality Management for the Twenty-First Century*. Tampa, FL: American College of Physician Executives; 1991:331–357.
37. Stover SL. Personal communication, 1994.
38. Stover SL. Spinal cord injury: Knowns and unknowns. *J Am Paraplegia Soc* 1993;17:1–6.
39. Johnston MV, Findley TW, DeLuca J, Katz RT. Research in physical medicine and rehabilitation: Measurement tools with application to brain injury. *Am J Phys Med Rehab* 1991;70:40–56.
40. Ruff RM, Marshall LF, Crouch J, Klauber MR, Levin HS, Barth J, Kreutzer J, Blunt BA, Foulkes MA, Eisenberg HM, Jane JA, Marmarou A. Predictors of outcome following severe head trauma. Follow-up data from the Traumatic Coma Databank. *Brain Inj* 1993;7:101–111.
41. Rappaport M, Hall KM, Hopkins K, Belleza T, Cope DN. Disability rating scale for severe head trauma: Coma to community. *Arch Phys Med Rehabil* 1982;63:118–123.
42. Schalock RL, Kiernen WE, McGaughey MJ, Lynch SA, McNally LC. State MR/DD agency information systems and available data related to day and employment programs. *Mental Retard* 1993;31:29–34.
43. Evans CD, Gibson J, Jones T, Williams MJ. A medical diagnostic index for rehabilitation. *Disability Rehab* 1993;15:127–135.
44. Gender AR. Developing and computerizing a patient classification system in a rehabilitation nursing setting. *Rehab Nurs* 1989;14:58–63.

45. McLaughlin K, Taylor S, Bliss-Holtz J, Sayres P, Nickle L. Shaping the future: The marriage of nursing theory and informatics. *Comput Nurs* 1990;8:174–179.

46. Orem D. *Nursing: Concepts of Practice*, 3rd ed. New York: McGraw-Hill; 1985.

47. Rudman D, McCormack J, Cuisinier M, Mattson DE. A simple method to quantify the changes in activities of daily living of long-stay nursing home populations. *Am J Phys Med Rehabil* 1993;72:276–280.

48. Zimny NJ, Tandy CJ. Development of a computer-assisted method for the collection, organization, and use of patient health history information in physical therapy. *J Sports Phys Ther* 1993;17:84–89.

49. Farrell WJ, Muik PA. Computer applications of streamline test scoring and other procedures and occupational therapy. *Am J Occup Ther* 1993;47:162–165.

50. Soede M. The use of information technology in rehabilitation: An overview of possibilities and new directions in applications. *J Med Eng Technol* 1989;13:5–9.

51. Lim I, Walkup R, Vannier MW. Rapid prototyping of interactive software for automated instrumentation in rehabilitative therapy. *Biomed Instrum Technol* 1992;26:209–214.

52. Milner M. Rehabilitation technology: Exploitation of R&D in current technologies. *Int J Rehabil Res* 1993;16:253–263.

53. New Abilities Systems, Inc. New Abilities USC 1000 with Tongue Touch Keypad. Palo Alto, CA: New Abilities Systems; 1994.

54. Faulkner VW, Walsh NE. Computer designed prosthetic socket from analysis of computer tomography data. *J Prosthet Orthoped* 1989;1(3):154–164.

55. Walsh NE, Lancaster JL, Faulkner VW, Rogers WE. A computerized system to manufacture prostheses for amputees in developing countries. *J Prosthet Orthoped* 1989;1(3):165–181.

56. Parkview Regional Rehabilitation Center, Fort Wayne, IN: Personal communication, 1994.

57. Hutzebiler T. Personal communication, 1994.

58. McDonald CJ, Barnett GO. Medical-record stored systems. In: Shortliffe EH, Perreault LE, eds. *Medical Informatics: Computer Applications in Health Care.* Reading, MA: Addison-Wesley; 1990:189–190.

59. Siegel ER, Cummings MM, Woodsmall RM. Bibliographic-retrieval services. In: Shortliffe EH, Perreault LE, eds. *Medical Informatics: Computer Applications in Health Care.* Reading, MA: Addison-Wesley; 1990:434–465.

60. Albright RG. *A Basic Guide to On-line Information Systems for Health Care Professionals.* Arlington, VA: Information Resource Press; 1992.

61. Roberts D. Coverage by four information services of the core journals of rehabilitation and related topics. *Scand J Rehab Med* 1992;24:167–173.

62. Davis J, Findley R. *Disability Rehab* 1993;15:127–135.

63. Wood MS, Horik EB, Snow B, eds. *End User Searching in the Health Sciences.* New York: Hayworth Press; 1986.

64. Broering NC. The Mini Medline system: A library-based end user search system. *Bull Med Libr Assoc* 1985;73:138–145.

65. Horowitz GL, Jackson JD, Bleich HL. Paperchase: Self-service bibliographic retrieval. *JAMA* 1983;250:2494–2499.

66. Sewell W. Overview of end user searching in the health sciences. In: Wood MS, Horrick EB, Snow B, eds. *End User Searching in the Health Sciences.* New York: Haywood Press; 1986:3–14.

67. Bohannon RW. Letter to the editor. *Am J Phys Med Rehabil* 1989;68:257.
68. Pollack R, ed. Computer network for disabled. *Traumagram* 1994;19:9.
69. Wiederhold G, Perreault LE. Hospital information systems. In: Shortliffe EH, Perreault LE, eds. *Medical Informatics: Computer Applications in Health Care.* Reading, MA: Addison-Wesley; 1990.
70. Friedman BA, Martin JB. Hospital information systems: The physicians' role. *JAMA* 1987;257:1792.

Section III

8
Trauma Registry Data Definition, Acquisition, and Evaluation

LINDA C. DEGUTIS

As information technology advances and data systems evolve, there is an opportunity to improve trauma registries and information systems within the broader context of the health information environment. Taking a proactive stance on the further development and improvement of trauma registries will allow for input into the design of health information technologies that can be utilized in the implementation of the registries.

Solomon et al., in a discussion of public health registries, noted that there are numerous considerations in registry implementation.[1] Since trauma registries are used to evaluate trauma care, assess effectiveness of trauma systems, and function as tools for research as well as determination of resource utilization,[2] this chapter focuses on the definition, acquisition, and evaluation of data to meet these needs. Issues of cost, integration with other data systems, optimal utilization of trauma registries in institutional and regional systems of trauma care, and the impact of technology on the future of trauma registries are also presented. Important points are illustrated with examples from the development of both hospital-based and statewide trauma registries.

The discussion in this chapter is based on several assumptions and definitions. "Trauma registry" refers to a data system that has been created either in an institution or on a regional level, with the primary purpose of evaluation of trauma care. "Region" refers to a geographic area that contains more than one institution that contributes data to a multi-institutional registry. "Trauma center" refers to an institution that has been verified as meeting trauma center criteria established by the American College of Surgeons or has been designated as a trauma center by a governmental body. "Trauma registrar" is defined as the person responsible for the collection and entry of data for the trauma registry, regardless of whether this is the formal title of the individual performing this function. The terms "data element," "data point," and "variable" are used interchangeably to designate a piece of data that is collected or calculated as part of the trauma data system. "Trauma patient" describes a patient who requires hospital-based treatment for injuries.

It is important to remember that trauma registries are widely variable in their data elements, case entry criteria, and methods of data collection and entry. While these differences may not necessarily affect the development of individual institutional registries, they do have a significant effect when multi-institutional registries are being considered.

Steps in Trauma Registry Data Definition

The definition of data points and data elements for use in a trauma data system is an important aspect of system development. This process involves multiple steps that include identification of potential users of the data, definition of the purpose of the data system, case criteria for entry into the data set, determination of the questions that will be asked of the data, determination of the data elements that will be collected to answer the questions, and definition of the data elements that will be collected.[3]

Identifying Users of the Data

Potential users of trauma data include clinicians, administrators, researchers, insurance providers, governmental agencies, and community agencies. These are defined in the broad sense, with clinicians ranging from emergency medical service providers to rehabilitation specialists who are involved in the care of trauma patients. Administrators include not only hospital and other institutional administrators, but also those who are responsible for managing or monitoring trauma systems and system components. Hospital administrators may be interested in evaluating the financial impact of trauma care on their institution. If they are providing funding for the registry, they will also have an interest in the cost of maintaining the data system, as well as the benefit of the system to their institution. Trauma system administrators will want to ensure that the registry contains data points necessary for system monitoring and evaluation. Insurance providers will be interested in outcomes and the cost of care for their clients. Multiple community agencies may have an interest in trauma data, since these bodies have responsibility for development of interventions and prevention programs that can have an impact on the occurrence of injuries. Governmental agencies such as local and state health departments may have an interest not only in the impact of a trauma system, but also in the effect of injuries on the population. It is important to define the potential users of the data prior to system development to permit informed decisions about data element inclusion and definition to be made with input from those who will be using the database.[4]

Define the Purpose of the Data System

Although the traditional purpose of trauma registries has been to monitor the quality of trauma care, as more potential users become familiar with the availability of registry data and aware of the potential for integration of the data with other data systems, more purposes will be identified. This trend will benefit the development of trauma data systems, since the justification for their existence will grow from that of utilization by a very small group of people to that of information needed by multiple groups, both within and outside an institution.

Potential uses of trauma registry data include quality improvement, outcomes research, injury epidemiology, injury surveillance, clinical research, trend analysis, and evaluation of resource utilization. Regional databases are likely to be used for trauma system evaluation as well as for epidemiology and surveillance.

If a decision is made to define a system that will meet the needs of multiple users, the needs of these users must be understood. Input from potential data users will provide the basis for building a comprehensive, usable system. A core group that represents the interests of users from various areas and multiple levels of database knowledge can serve the purpose of soliciting input from others who will use the data.

On a regional level, data are more likely to be used for system evaluation and planning, rather than for evaluation of individual cases. Data may also be used in the development of benchmarks for system and institutional performance. System administrators as well as institutions involved in the system will have an interest in examining aggregate data for purposes of comparison multi-institutional performance and evaluation of trauma system issues. In addition, the development of a multi-institutional database, entails multiple costs, especially if the purpose differs from that of similar databases at the participating institutions. Institutions may have to modify or restructure their own data sets to provide the information needed for the regional registry. This all comes at a cost. It is therefore important to include representatives of these groups when planning the registry.

Determine What Questions Will Be Asked of the Data

Before data elements can be defined, it is necessary to determine what questions will be asked of the data. Forethought in this area will help to define the scope and complexity of the data system that is set up. It will also provide a definition of the data elements to be included in the data set. It is important to keep in mind that some questions will need to be asked on a consistent basis, and others will need to be asked only periodically or only once. To support a study of trends in utilization of hospital resources such as critical care beds, for example, the registry must contain data that will allow for the determination of length of patient stay in the intensive care unit (ICU). If other ICU resource parameters are to be measured on a continuous basis, data elements related to these must also be included.

With respect to prevention activities, a program planner might be interested in learning more about the types of injury events that occur in a specific community and whether members of the community use protective devices such as seat belts and helmets. In addition, clusters of injury outbreaks in the community can be identified, much as outbreaks of infectious diseases are identified. Risk factors for injury can be explored, provided there is detail about these risks in the data set.

Questions related to physiologic parameters (e.g., lowest blood pressure each day in the ICU) are rarely asked of the data on a regular basis. Clinicians and quality improvement personnel are likely to be interested in knowing the Revised Trauma Score[5] for a large number of patients in the registry, however, because when this information is combined with other data elements such as age and the Injury Severity Score,[6] it can be used in predicted mortality studies. Clearly, it is also important to understand the components of these two scores, so that the appropriate data points can be collected for the calculation of the scores.

Questions related to specific issues that are not expected to be of long-standing duration should not be considered when the scope of the database is being defined. What should be considered in this context is the nature of the questions that are likely to be asked on an ad hoc or one-time basis, so that options for periodic collection of data elements needed to answer time-limited questions can be created.

On a regional level, there may be a desire to use the trauma data system for injury surveillance activities. As noted earlier, clusters of injury occurrence can be identified and interventions developed to prevent further clusters. For example, if three adolescents in the same town were killed in separate motor vehicle crashes within a month, the data system could be used not only to identify this cluster, but to pinpoint the location of each event, and to determine whether environmental factors contributed to the crashes, whether alcohol or drugs may have been a factor, whether protective devices were used, and whether neighboring towns experienced the same problem. In addition, it would be possible to measure the effectiveness of interventions that were implemented by observing additional events after the interventions were put into place.

Trends and patterns in injury occurrence for a specific area or region can be monitored using a well-designed trauma data set. The data system would have to be inclusive, to provide a true picture of persons who are injured. If there is a desire to use the trauma data system for the purpose of surveillance as described here, it is necessary to ensure that all cases of injury will be included.

Determine What Data Elements Will Be Collected

Since the number and type of data elements collected will have a great impact on the cost and effectiveness of the data system, it is crucial to devote much time and thought to this aspect of the registry and data system development. Keep in mind that there is a cost associated with the collection of each data element. This cost is determined by the ease of collection of the data element, the complexity of the data element, and the time it takes to code and enter the data element. There should be justification for the inclusion of each data point that is to be collected. That is, it should be clear that any data elements collected will be used on a regular basis by at least one user of the data system. All data points should be relevant and necessary to answer the questions that will be asked of the system. It is easy to fall into the trap of collecting multiple data elements that "might be nice to have in case we want to look at . . .". There is no justification for using this rationale to include irrelevant or unnecessary data elements. In fact, by failing to screen proposed data elements, it is possible to come up with a duplication of the medical record, which is not what this type of data system is supposed to be. Rather, there is the opportunity to add or modify data elements on a regular basis, and any system should have a review process to allow this capability to be built into the system.

Data elements to be collected will fall into several categories: demographic data, prehospital data, injury event data, emergency department (ED) data, diagnostic study data, operating room data, ICU data, hospital ward data, diagnosis(es) and scoring data, discharge data, rehabilitation data, financial data, and system evaluation data. Examples of data elements in each of these categories appear in Table 8.1.

In the establishment of a regional data system, there are unique issues to be addressed. Consideration must be given to what type of data and what data elements are currently being collected by institutions and services in the region. If collecting data beyond these fields is clearly needed and justified, the issue of additional data collection cost and who will absorb the cost will have to be considered. There may also be a cost involved in modifying institutional and service databases to include new permanent fields, so the justification for these will need to be explicit.

Define the Data Elements That Are Being Collected

At first glance, it might appear that the definition of data elements would be easy. Ease of definition is deceptive, however, and there are numerous considerations in developing the data element definition. For data elements that are commonly used by multiple systems, it is important to have consistency in definition. Data elements must be described concisely, but with enough detail that the definitions are clear. That is, the description of a data element should be supplemented by documentation of its meaning. In

TABLE 8.1. Categories of data elements

Category	Example
Demographic	Age, gender, residence address, ethnicity
Prehospital	Time of EMS arrival on scene, blood pressure, pulse, respiratory rate
Injury event	Location of event, text description of event, protective device use
Emergency department	ED interventions, blood pressure, pulse, respiratory rate, GCS
Diagnostic studies	CT scan date, time and results, x-rays performed
Operating room	Operative procedures, date(s) and time(s) of operations, surgeon
ICU	Dates of admission and discharge from ICU; ICU procedures (bronchoscopy, tube thoracostomy, etc.)
Hospital ward	Dates of admission and discharge from ward
Diagnosis(es) and scoring	Text description of injuries, information for calculation of Glasgow Coma Score, Revised Trauma Score, Injury Severity Score
Discharge	Date of discharge from hospital, status at time of discharge, place discharged to
Rehabilitation	Name of rehabilitation facility, functional status at admission and at discharge from rehab
Financial	Payer source, charges, reimbursement
System evaluation	EMS dispatch and arrival times, triage criteria used, trauma team notification and arrival times

addition, it is useful to identify the location of the data element in the original source document.

For calculated data fields, it is essential that the definition be clear about exactly which data elements will be used in the calculation. The Revised Trauma Score for in-hospital use is calculated from the systolic blood pressure, the score on the Glasgow Coma Score (GCS),[7] and the respiratory rate at a given time. Since there may be several records of these measurements, it is important to state which should be used for the calculation. This must be clear not only to the person who is collecting the data but also to the data users.

If there are local, regional, or national standards for coding of data elements, it is important that the trauma data system's coding scheme match these standards. Definitions of data points may be made easier by the use of some of these standards. It is common to use the International Classification of Diseases (ICD) nomenclature for coding of injury events (external cause of injury: E-codes) as well as injury diagnosis(es) (nature of injury: N-codes). The limitations of these codes should also be understood, especially if it is anticipated that the codes will be used to determine injury severity.

A record of the data element definitions, or data dictionary (Table 8.2) should be maintained. This will help to avoid confusion about the meaning

TABLE 8.2. Data dictionary structure

Date element	Definition
Injury event (text)	A text description of the event that resulted in the patient's injury. This description should include as much detail as possible about the circumstances of the event. For all injuries, it is important to include information that assists in defining the amount of energy that was transmitted (e.g., height from which patient fell, speed of motor vehicle, patient location in vehicle). For intentional injuries, additional information should be included about the assailant (relationship to patient), type of weapon used, and circumstances leading to the assault. Source: prehospital run form, ED triage note, trauma team admission notes Field size: 255 characters Field type: text Mandatory field: yes Index field: no Field used for calculation of other data points: no Default value: none Missing data value: "information not available"
Prehospital blood pressure	The initial blood pressure that is measured when EMS providers arrive at the scene. Source: prehospital run form Field size: 3 Field type: integer Mandatory field: yes (if patient was transported by EMS) Index field: no Field used for calculation of other data points: yes (Revised Trauma Score) Default value: none Missing data value: -1
Glasgow Coma Score from emergency department	The GCS measured at the time the patient arrives in the ED, based on the three measures that constitute the GCS: eye opening, verbal response, and motor response Source: calculated field (from ED values) or direct entry from nurse's notes Field size: 2 Field type: integer Mandatory field: no Index field: no Field used for calculation of other data points: yes (Revised Trauma Score) Default value: none Missing data value: -1

of specific pieces of data. The data dictionary should include the specific definition of each data element, as well as descriptive information about the configuration (size, format, calculation if applicable) of the data element. In addition, it is helpful to include the location of the data element in the original source document.

Develop Data Linkage Strategies

Many data elements may already be available in other data systems that can be integrated or linked with the trauma database. Creating linkages can lead to significant cost savings by eliminating the need to make duplicate entries of data elements that are already available; the potential for errors in data input may be decreased, as well. Data are usually linked through the use of unique identifiers, such as medical record number, that are available in each of the data sets being linked.

It may be necessary to use a combination of a unique identifier with one or two other variables to ensure that the data items being linked are those that are desired. The following case example illustrates the importance of this. John G. is the 62-year-old driver of a car that was involved in a motor vehicle crash on May 26, 1996. He experienced a brief loss of consciousness at the scene of the crash but was awake and alert with a GCS of 15 at the time of his arrival in the ED. A computed tomography (CT) scan of the patient's head, performed at the time of his ED visit, was interpreted to be normal, and Mr. G. was discharged. On May 28, 1996, however, he returned to the ED with a decreased level of consciousness (GCS 11) and a history of a seizure at home. Another head CT scan was performed, which showed a subdural hematoma. Upon further investigation, it was discovered that the patient had fallen at home earlier in the day, hitting his head against a wall.

The trauma registrar uses information from the diagnostic imaging database as part of the trauma registry. Each patient in the hospital is assigned a unique medical record number that is used whenever that patient visits the hospital for diagnostic studies or treatment. Using the medical record number only, for linking the data, the results of John G.'s first CT scan might be added to the trauma registry data set. Adding the ED visit date as another linkage tool, it is possible to ensure that the first CT scan reading, which is copied to the registry data set, accompanies the scan from the second visit.

The linkage of data with external data sets presents additional problems. The probabilistic method of data linkage utilizes multiple identifiers that may appear in more than one data set and can be used to approach 100% accuracy in identifying cases. This method takes the identifiers that are most likely to match between the data sets and searches for matches. Once a match has been made, a secondary identifier is matched to improve the probability that the same cases are being identified in each of the data sets. This procedure may be continued for several data elements to provide the optimal chance of an accurate link. A criterion for linkage is established, in that it may be decided that if there is a match between the first three identifiers, the data will be linked and the case record completed. The CODES [Crash Outcome Data Evaluation System] projects[8] that were funded by the National Highway Traffic Safety Administration (NHTSA) demonstrated this method for linking data from multiple sources in studies aimed at assessing the effectiveness of vehicle occupant protection measures. A more detailed discussion of data linkage is beyond the scope of this chapter. The reader is referred to reports from the CODES projects[9] as well as to articles by Clark,[10] Copes et al.,[11] Langley and Botha,[12] Muse et al.,[13] and Shevchencko et al.[14]

Another difficulty with data linkage is evident when cases of interest do not appear in each of the data sets being linked. Not all motor vehicle crashes are reported to the police, even when injuries result.[15] Because of the absence of such cases from police records, important information about these crashes is not available.

It is important to determine whether there are methods in place for ensuring the accuracy of data that are obtained from secondary sources. This is a more important issue with some data elements than with others. For example, if laboratory data are stored in a database, having selected lab values downloaded to a trauma database would be more effective than requiring users to extract values individually from the medical record. The fewer the occasions for data to pass through human hands, the less chance there is for data entry error.

There are, however, data elements that are problematic with respect to transfer from one database to another. This is true for the nature-of-injury codes (N-codes) from the ninth revision of the ICD (ICD-9), since there is a great deal of opportunity for variation in determining the codes that are assigned to the diagnoses for each patient. The trauma registrar may be very familiar with the use of N-codes related to injury and may feel comfortable with the utilization of these codes. The medical records coder or billing coder may be less familiar with the idiosyncrasies of the injury N-codes, especially with respect to coding for injury severity. In addition, at many institutions this function is not performed by a single coder, so there is likely to be more variability in the way that N-codes are assigned. A similar difficulty exists with respect to E-codes, which can be difficult to assign based on the information that is available in a given patient's record.

Determine How the Data Will Be Collected and Stored

Issues that need to be addressed include prospective versus retrospective data abstraction and data entry, paper versus paperless methods of data collection, and local versus network or mainframe data entry and storage. Prospective data collection allows for more detail and potentially more accuracy in the data set, since there is an opportunity to ask questions about what is meant by entries in the medical record. This method is more labor intensive than a retrospective review of the data, but it is important to remember that prospective data entry offers other benefits. In the course of abstracting and entering the data, it is possible to note the absence of essential data items, identify quality of care issues early enough to ensure timely interventions, and monitor the record for completeness and timeliness of record entries.

Paperless modes of data collection, such as direct data entry into a laptop or desktop computer, decrease the time needed to enter each record, since data are recorded only once, rather than being copied onto a paper form and then entered into a computer. Scannable forms are available, which can be scanned into the database once data have been entered. Prehospital care providers are the most frequent users of scannable forms.

Data that are collected should be backed up on a regular basis. This may be easiest if the data are stored on a network computer, but to maintain patient confidentiality, provisions must be made for data security. Multiple levels of security are available; for example, some software programs allow only specified users to modify or view data of certain types.

Determine Who Will Be Responsible for Collecting the Data, as Well as Who Will Be Responsible for Ensuring Accuracy of the Data

To ensure that the database functions optimally, it is necessary to clearly delineate responsibilities for data collection, data entry, data linkages, uploads/downloads, and data quality. The need for accuracy in data extraction and entry cannot be overstressed. Reports based on the data will be only as good as the quality of the data that are entered. Mechanisms should be developed for monitoring the quality of the data regularly, through the use of spot checks of data fields and data records. It is possible and highly desirable to build data checks into the software that is used to maintain the data. Even if this is done, routine manual checks of data should be performed to identify areas in which there are problems.

Determine Who Will Have Access to the Data and How That Access Will Be Provided

Users of the trauma data will require varying levels of access. Direct access to the database, with the ability to modify records or alter the database, should be limited to those who will be performing data entry and data quality functions. Other access to the data should generally be restricted to certain portions of the data set or be provided in the form of data reports regularly furnished to users who require them. Those who use the data for research purposes may be allowed to download needed data elements to a separate file for use in the investigation.

To provide this type of functionality of the data set with respect to report design and generation and data downloads, it is important that the persons working with the database understand and be able to interpret the needs of the users who are requesting the data. In addition, the users should be provided with clear explanations of what is and is not available from the data set, as well as definitions of the variables that are being reported.

Determine Which Reports Will Be Needed on a Regular Basis

Reports based on data in the trauma registry can take numerous forms. Routine reports may be used for many purposes, such as monitoring the number and type of patients admitted to the hospital, tracking trends in injury severity and outcome, monitoring predetermined quality improvement measures, and evaluating trends in resource utilization. It should be determined regularly what data are needed, and reports should be designed to meet these needs. It is generally very straightforward to program these report templates into the database so that documents can be easily generated.

Traditionally, trauma registry data have not been well utilized for the purposes of studying injury epidemiology and planning and evaluating injury prevention interventions. There is good reason for this, insofar as inherent biases in trauma registry data create problems with the application to the population as a whole of conclusions based on such specialized data. Trauma registries have traditionally consisted of data on a select set of patients who are admitted to a select group of institutions. The biases in these registries are toward the inclusion of persons who are most seriously injured and are most likely to be transported to trauma centers. Each institution has its own criteria for inclusion in the registry database, with a large group of institutions including only cases that meet criteria for trauma center triage, trauma team activation, or admission to a trauma service. In addition, data collected as part of a trauma registry are often collected primarily for quality improvement or system development purposes and may not include information necessary for performing epidemiologic studies of injury.

Trauma registry data can be useful in planning and evaluation of trauma care, as well as the planning and evaluation of trauma prevention programs. For example, it is possible to estimate the magnitude of trauma occurrence within a specific area to plan for health care services that should be provided, as well as to determine the need for interventions to prevent specific types of injury within a community.

Surveillance of injuries within a given area is also important. As Lloyd and Graitcer point out, trauma registries do have a potential use in injury surveillance.[16] Again, a regional registry can provide information about clusters of injuries, such as those that might be attributable to the use of snowblowers during the first snowstorm of the season, or injuries due to fireworks over the Fourth of July weekend. Obviously, the selection of cases for inclusion in the registry has a significant effect on whether this will be possible a given community. When registries are used for surveillance, inherent biases in the data must be kept in mind. As Payne and Waller have suggested, a major restructuring of trauma registries is necessary if they are to be useful for documenting and studying the problem of injury.[17]

Data that are frequently lacking or minimal in trauma registries are the data points that are often most helpful in studying causes of injury. It is often difficult to find information specific to assailants or type of weapon used in cases of interpersonal violence. Directions of vehicular impact, as well as forces causing injury, often are not available.[18,19] Protective device use is often recorded with respect to motor vehicle–related injuries, but it is documented less often in injury events associated with sports or recreational activities. The use of alcohol or other drugs in proximity to an injury event is not always tested for or documented. Many of these data are missing because they are not available in the medical record. Despite these issues, the trauma registry can provide essential data not found in other data sets. As with any database, it is important to realize the limitations of the data included and to take these limitations into consideration when using the data.[20]

The literature contains examples of the use of trauma registries, especially those that are hospital based, for research,[21–23] quality improvement,[24–27] and trauma system evaluation,[28,29] as well as for surveillance[30] and epidemiology.[31] In addition, a number of these papers document the importance of data linkages to form a more comprehensive picture of injury occurrence.

Data System Evaluation

Benefits

One question that must be answered with respect to trauma data systems is: How do they benefit the institution or region? The answer to this question will aid in justifying the resource commitment required to maintain the data sets. Some potential benefits to an institution, other than the ability to maintain trauma center verification and/or designation, include ability to monitor quality improvement activities, assessment of resource utilization by injured patients, and monitoring trends in patient care.

Regional data systems can be beneficial in monitoring a newly developed trauma system, providing population-based data on the injury problem, and evaluating the effectiveness of programmatic interventions. Each of these functions will depend on the data system structure and the needs of the data users.

Costs

In addition to the cost of personnel salaries for the maintenance of the database, costs that must be considered include software, computer hardware, software support and upgrades, and training. When a system is to be extended beyond an institution, it is necessary to determine whether the costs of maintaining the system will be absorbed by the institutions that contribute data or passed on to external users. These costs should clearly be considered in the initial design of the database, as well as in periodic evaluations of the data system.

Review Data Elements

Data elements should be reviewed to determine their continued utility and to recommend new data elements far more frequent than is typically done. The addition of data elements should not be taken lightly, and there should be sufficient justification for adding any data elements that will require more collection time and effort. New data elements should be evaluated in much the same way as initial data elements in a new database are evaluated. Often, variables that are collected are rarely, if ever, used. Again, the need for a regular review of data elements should help to eliminate extraneous data points. This practice will also decrease data entry and collection time.

Review Reports

Regularly generated reports should be reviewed for their utility. Users of the reports should be asked to provide feedback, including suggestions for improving the documents. It may be necessary to modify the database to address user concerns, but again there should be a clear justification for making changes.

State and Regional Data Systems

Data systems at the state and regional levels differ from hospital-based registries in that they are more likely to require complex data linkages and may provide population-based assessment of the injury problem. The design of these systems should follow essentially the same steps as the design of hospital-based registries, especially the inclusion of interested and affected parties in the system development. It is especially important to include persons who are knowledgeable about data collection, data definition, and evaluation, as well as clinical issues.

State trauma registries have been utilized for promotion of prevention activities, development of legislation, and trauma system evaluation.[32] Often, hospital discharge data sets are used to define and study the injury problem on a regional basis. This approach is not without problems, since the discharge data sets may include many cases (e.g., readmissions for further treatment of an injury) that would not be considered in the calculation of true hospital admission incidence rates.[33] Many states do not require that hospital discharge data contain E-codes, which would be of great benefit in examining hospitalizations for incidence of injury.[34]

Using New Technology and New Processes

The potential for development of an electronic medical record (EMR) opens up new opportunities for trauma registry growth. The EMR has yet to become a reality for many reasons. As Carpenter points out, there are a number of probable barriers to the development of a comprehensive data system, including human interface with computer systems, system performance (with particular reference to speed, speech recognition technology, infrastructure of network systems, and processing of text information), confidentiality and security issues, and common standards for data.[35]

Development of technology that allows remote data entry through the Internet will enhance the ability to link multiple data sets as well as multi-institutional databases. The technology is available but has yet to be developed or utilized to its fullest potential.

Summary

Careful selection of data points and attention to what will be used and needed are essential in the development of trauma registries. Once structured, no registry should be viewed as completed, but should be reviewed regularly to ensure that data collection is accurate and that the system provides the data that are needed in a cost-effective manner. As new technology becomes available, the potential for more efficient and useful trauma data systems will grow. It will be important to ensure that trauma registries do not become duplications of the medical record. Rather, they must be defined in such a way that they serve the purposes for which they were intended during initial design and regular evaluation phases.

References

1. Solomon DJ, Henry RC, Hogan JG, Van Amburg GH, Taylor J. Evaluation and implementation of public health registries. *Public Health Rep* 1991;106:142–150.

2. Pollock DA, McClain PW. Trauma registries: Current status and future prospects. *JAMA* 1989;262:2280–2283.
3. Pollock DA, McClain PW. Report from the 1988 Trauma Registry Workshop, including recommendations for hospital-based trauma registries. *J Trauma* 1989;29:827–834.
4. Sheps S. Components of a minimum data set. *Can J Public Health* 1989;80:430–432.
5. Champion HR, Sacco WJ, Copes WS, Gann DS, Gennarelli TA, Flanagan ME. A revision of the Trauma Score. *J Trauma* 1989;29:623–629.
6. Baker SP, O'Neill B, Haddon W, Long WB. The Injury Severity Score: A method for describing patients with multiple injuries and evaluating emergency care. *J Trauma* 1974;14:187–196.
7. Teasdale G, Jennett B. Assessment of coma and impaired consciousness: A practical scale. *Lancet* 1974;2:81–84.
8. National Highway Traffic Safety Administration. The Crash Outcome Data Evaluation System (CODES). DOT HS 808 338. National Technical Information Service, Technical Report. Springfield, VA: NHTSA; 1996.
9. National Highway Traffic Safety Administration. Benefits of Safety Belts and Motorcycle Helmets: Report to Congress, February 1996. Washington, DC: U.S. Department of Transportation; 1996.
10. Clark DE. Development of a statewide trauma registry using multiple linked sources of data. *AMIA* 1994;1:654–658.
11. Copes WS, Stark MM, Lawnick MM, Teper S, Wilderson D, DeJong G, Brannon R, Hamilton BB. Linking data from national trauma and rehabilitation registries. *J Trauma* 1996;40:428–436.
12. Langley JD, Botha JL. Use of record linkage techniques to maintain the Leicestershire Diabetes Register. *Comp Methods Prog Biomed* 1994;41:287–295.
13. Muse AG, Mikl J, Smith PF. Evaluating the quality of anonymous record linkage using deterministic procedures with the New York State AIDS Registry and a hospital discharge file. *Stat Med* 1995;14:499–509.
14. Shevchenko IP, Lynch JT, Mattie AS, Reed-Fourquet LL. Verification of information in a large medical database using linkages with external databases. *Stat Med* 1995;14:511–530.
15. Rosman DL, Knuiman MW. A comparison of hospital and police road injury data. *Accident Anal Prev* 1994;26:215–222.
16. Lloyd LE, Graitcer PL. The potential for using a trauma registry for injury surveillance and prevention. *Am J Prev Med* 1989;5:34–37.
17. Payne SR, Waller JA. Trauma registry and trauma center biases in injury research. *J Trauma* 1989;29:424–429.
18. Santana JR, Martinez R. Accuracy of emergency physician data collection in automobile collisions. *J Trauma* 1995;38:583–586.
19. Waller JA. Methodologic issues in hospital-based injury research. *J Trauma* 1988;28:1632–1636.
20. Kuller LH. The use of existing databases in morbidity and mortality studies. *Am J Public Health* 1995;85:1198–1199.
21. Champion HR, Copes WS, Sacco WJ, Lawnick MM, Keast SL, Bain LW, Flanagan ME, Frey CF. The Major Trauma Outcome Study: Establishing national norms for trauma care. *J Trauma* 1990;30:1356–1365.

22. Sacco WJ, Copes WS, Bain LW, MacKenzie EJ, Frey CF, Hoyt DB, Weigelt JA, Champion HR. Effect of preinjury illness on trauma patient survival outcome. *J Trauma* 1993;35:538–543.

23. Kizer KW, Vassar MJ, Harry RL, Layton KD. Hospitalization charges, costs, and income for firearm-related injuries at a university trauma center. *JAMA* 1995;273:1768–1773.

24. Nayduch D, Moylan J, Snyder BL, Andrews L, Rutledge R, Cunningham P. American College of Surgeons trauma quality indicators: An analysis of outcome in a statewide trauma registry. *J Trauma* 1994;37:565–575.

25. Karmy-Jones R, Copes WS, Champion HR, Weigelt J, Shackford S, Lawnick M, Roszycki GS, Hollingsworth-Fridlund P, Klein J. Results of a multi-institutional outcome assessment: Results of a structured peer review of TRISS-designated unexpected outcomes. *J Trauma* 1992;35:196–203.

26. Vestrup JA, Phang T, Vertesi L, Wing PC, Hamilton NE. The utility of a multicenter regional trauma registry. *J Trauma* 1994;37:375–378.

27. Copes WS, Staz CF, Konvalinka CW, Sacco WJ. American College of Surgeons audit filters: Associations with patient outcome and resource utilization. *J Trauma* 1995;38:432–438.

28. Stewart TC, Lane PL, Stefanits T. An evaluation of patient outcomes before and after trauma center designation using trauma and injury severity score analysis. *J Trauma* 1995;39:1036–1040.

29. Kane G, Wheeler NC, Cook S, Engelhardt R, Pavey B, Green K, Clark ON, Cassou J. Impact of the Los Angeles Country trauma system on the survival of seriously injured patients. *J Trauma* 1992;32:576–583.

30. Orsay E, Holden JA, Williams J, Lumpkin JR. Motorcycle trauma in the State of Illinois: Analysis of the Illinois Department of Public Health Trauma Registry. *Ann Emerg Med* 1995;26:455–460.

31. Woodruff BA, Baron RC. A description of nonfatal spinal cord injury using a hospital-based registry. *Am J Prev Med* 1994;10:10–14.

32. Shapiro MJ, Cole KE, Keegan M, Prasad CN, Thompson RJ. National survey of state trauma registries—1992. *J Trauma* 1994;37:835–842.

33. Smith GS, Langlois JA, Buechner JS. Methodological issues in using hospital discharge data to determine the incidence of hospitalized injuries. *Am J Epidemiol* 1991;134:1146–1158.

34. Sniezek JE, Finklea JF, Graitcer PL. Injury coding and hospital discharge data. *JAMA* 1989;262:2270–2272.

35. Carpenter PC. The electronic medical record: Perspective from Mayo Clinic. *Int J Bio-Med Comput* 1994;34:159–171.

9
Trauma Registry Informatics: Hospital Perspectives

Sheryl Zougras, Thomas J. Esposito, and Kimball I. Maull

The provision of trauma care is a complex endeavor that is highly dependent on collection of data that should be converted into useful information. The data collected come from a variety of sources, including the patient, the prehospital setting and providers, the emergency department, other acute care hospital venues, and the post–acute care setting. These data attempt to track the care of the patient on the continuum that begins at the scene of the injury and ends with the patient's death or final postinjury level of recovery and function in society. Furthermore, many parties interested in health care and injury control, both within and outside the hospital, will find the information provided by a hospital database useful.

Efforts to care for the patient must be coordinated and integrated. Likewise, the management and analysis of patient care data must be coordinated and integrated to permit evaluation of the results and the effectiveness of care.

Because of the importance of the data and information just described, a specific entity, the trauma registry, has evolved in many hospitals caring for injured patients. The trauma registry can serve to identify strengths and deficiencies of care, provide the necessary impetus to effect change, and therefore play a part in improving the quality and value of patient care. These attributes should make the trauma registry and its staff an integral component of the trauma team and a valuable resource.

The ultimate goal of a hospital trauma registry is to acquire, manage, and use information to enhance and improve individual provider, institutional, and system performance as well as patient care and outcome. The efficiency and effectiveness of the information management process may well be affected by the technologies employed. However, the success or failure of the trauma registry ultimately depends on the commitment of the hospital and its staff. Successful trauma data management is also related to concise, clearly defined objectives and inclusion criteria, the data elements collected, and the presence of an established mechanism to assess and maintain the integrity of the data, then analysis, and proper use.

Trauma Registry Objectives

The existence of a hospital trauma registry may initially stem from the hospital's desire to maintain designation or accreditation by regulatory agencies. However, the greater purpose and mission of a trauma registry should be multifaceted. The objectives of a hospital trauma registry may include, but not be limited to, developing, implementing, and evaluating systems of trauma care. This can apply within the hospital and its immediate catchment area or as part of a larger regional or state system of care. The hospital-based trauma registry is somewhat limited in this respect to issues related to prehospital care and acute hospital care. The main focus of most hospital-based trauma registries is facilitating hospital quality assurance and improvement, as well as compliance with trauma system standards where they exist. The hospital trauma registry can also be used to assess the performance of staff, the utilization of resources, and the cost effectiveness or value of the care provided. Furthermore, it can serve as a tool to aid in education or research as well as in injury epidemiology and surveillance. It can also serve as the foundation for identification, implementation, and evaluation of injury prevention strategies and programs. Finally, it can support public information and education as well as legislative initiatives.

Despite this robust potential, the trauma registry cannot effectively serve all these purposes equally. Each objective must be clearly defined and prioritized, with the focus being set by a medical director. These objectives and the focus of the registry will determine the role it plays in the hospital treating trauma patients and within the greater trauma system, where one exists. The most successful and useful trauma registries are those that have the capability through both programmatic direction and technology to serve multiple purposes, yet are flexible and adaptable to changes in focus over time.

Methods of Data Acquisition

To some degree the foregoing objectives will dictate the methods of data acquisition and review of patient records. Record review can be retrospective, concurrent, or a combination of both. Retrospective review conserves resources. It allows for all data to be retrieved, coded, and entered at one time. It will generally not allow for timely identification of trends and provider feedback.

Concurrent review requires a significant commitment of personnel. Charts may be reviewed at several junctures during a patient's hospital course. With this method, patients are diagnosed earlier, as are trends in care as well as complications. This allows more timely analysis and appropriate intervention. Provider behaviors or patient care issues can be addressed more effectively when interventions are instituted in closer temporal relationship to adverse occurrences. Concurrent data entry also facilitates prompt generation and dissemination of registry reports.

With a combined approach, using both retrospective and concurrent review, issues identified as needing immediate attention can be addressed in the appropriate time frame. Charts may be reviewed upon a patient's entry into the system, and then again after discharge. Charts of patients with intermediate or extended lengths of stay may be reviewed one or more times prior to discharge. Trends on certain parameters will be reported and followed based on the total number of patients admitted and discharged during a certain time frame. Quality of care issues addressed in this fashion (e.g., trends in nosocomial pneumonia or deep venous thrombosis) will affect future patients, not necessarily the patient currently hospitalized.

Ultimately, the method of record review will be selected on the basis of the objectives established for the trauma registry. The current trend is toward a more concurrent data management system. This allows for analysis of the care given today to affect management strategy and quality improvement issues tomorrow.

Inclusion Criteria

Database inclusion criteria must be concise and well defined. Currently, there is no standard and generally accepted definition of a trauma patient or a major trauma patient, much less consensus on which injured patients should be included in a trauma registry. Trauma patient definitions and trauma registry case inclusion criteria have been proposed or employed by some organizations. These include the American College of Surgeons (ACS), the Major Trauma Outcome Study (MTOS) database it sponsored, and Centers for Disease Control and Prevention (CDC).[1-3] Many hospital and state trauma system registries continue to use their own case inclusion criteria.

Most databases have conformed to the use of the ninth revision of the International Classification of Diseases (ICD-9) CM diagnostic injury codes to identify an injured patient, but not necessarily for inclusion in a trauma registry.[3,4] Traumatic injuries fall within codes 800 to 959.9, which refer to the specific nature of the disease or injury (i.e., the N-codes). An additional descriptor that has become important in identifying trauma patients in many databases is the external cause or etiology code (E-code).[5] The pertinent E-codes for trauma patients range between 800 and 999.

Many hospital trauma registries exclude drownings and poisonings. Inclusion of isolated hip fractures from low level falls has also been a point of controversy in considering inclusion criteria for some registries. Registries also differ considerably as to whether factors such as a patient's admission to the hospital, length of stay, need of intensive care, or Injury Severity Score (ISS) are accepted as part of the case inclusion criteria. Individual institutions or trauma systems often determine the inclusion criteria that pertain to their databases. This practice has implications for comparison of data between and within trauma systems and hospitals.

Serious consideration must be given to deciding on case inclusion criteria for the hospital trauma registry. First, the ability to query the database for specific patient populations will be affected by this decision. For example, the exclusion of patients with an ISS of less than 9 will not allow for reporting on all patients with traumatic pelvic fractures, since such an injury can result in an ISS ranging from 4 to 25.

Adjustment of inclusion criteria is also a factor in regulating the size and complexity of the database. Any change in the inclusion criteria should be noted, since these can change the number and nature of patients in the database and therefore the appearance of a hospital's trauma care profile. Such changes in an individual hospital's inclusion criteria or differences in inclusion criteria between two hospital registries may account for perceived changes or differences in resource utilization, volume, and costs. Therefore, it is important to consider these criteria when data from the registry are analyzed and conclusions drawn from the analyses.

Data Elements

Data element selection may be based on local, regional, state, or national considerations. Mandatory or voluntary reporting of data to certain regulatory and accrediting bodies such as a trauma system lead agency, the Joint Commission for the Accreditation of Healthcare Organizations (JCAHO) or the proposed National Trauma Data Bank of the American College of Surgeons, should be consider when data elements for the hospital registry are being selected. Any data elements necessary to fulfill external reporting obligations should serve as a template to which other elements are added. This will mitigate the need for duplicative data collection, entry, and submission efforts.

Additional data elements should be chosen with care. The data set and its size will influence the nature, scope, content, and integrity of potentially available information.[6] Each data element included should serve to help answer a question and should be easily measurable. Before any element is included in the database, the questions it will aid in answering should be determined. Collection merely for the sake of collection of data elements that are not useful will hamper the efficiency of the trauma registry. Overcollection adds to the time of chart abstracting and can diminish the accuracy and completeness of the registry database.

When designing a registry database, it is best to start with a small number of easily identifiable and capturable elements, which serve to provide the answers to a few important questions about trauma care at the hospital. Data sets packaged in a number of commercial software products may contain a large number of data elements. An individual trauma registry is not obligated to collect all of them, only those that are available and relevant. Most software product data sets can be modified either by the commercial supplier or by the user prior to or after installation. A small but pertinent database can be instituted and then expanded by the uses as the data acquisition and management process becomes more familiar. To begin with a large and unwieldy data set, on too large a patient population, generated by liberally set inclusion criteria, will undoubtedly doom a registry to failure at the outset.

It is imperative that each data element be concisely defined. A succinct data element dictionary will provide consistency in both data abstraction and proper interpretation of information gleaned from the collected data. A concisely defined data dictionary will reduce subjectivity in data abstraction and help mitigate inconsistencies based on variation in abstractor interpretation. The data dictionary should also provide information to the abstractor as to the primary source in the patient record from which each data element should be sought. It should indicate which data source is considered to be most reliable and acceptable. In addition, the data dictionary should provide direction as to when to leave a data field blank and when to indicate that an element was not documented or a test or procedure designed to yield the element was not done. The data set and data entry process should also allow for the discernment of these situations.

Several examples, cited to illustrate these points, clearly reveal how lack of standard definitions and abstracting policies and procedures can influence reliability and comparability of data abstracted by different abstractors or at different hospitals.

We begin with the data element "systolic blood pressure in the emergency department." Options for entry may include the first blood pressure appearing on the emergency department (ED) record, the lowest blood pressure, the highest blood pressure, or any blood pressure. This piece of data might be gleaned from various sources, including the nursing records and the physician's notes. To prevent uncertainty on these points, a clearly defined statement such as the following might appear in a published policy and procedure manual or data dictionary:

The systolic blood pressure in the emergency department is defined as the first blood pressure recorded on the nursing flow sheet after patient arrival in the ED. If this is not available, and ED initial blood pressure recorded in the physician's notes may suffice. If neither is documented, entry of the value 999 will denote this. If the patient had no obtainable blood pressure, the value of 000 should be entered.

Another example involving the Glasgow Coma Score (GCS) is also cogent. A policy might define a hierarchy of acceptable sources such as the following:

The initial GCS is that which is recorded in the ED on the nursing flow sheet. If not documented there, a GCS listed in the admission notes of the physician is acceptable. If neither of the above is present, the GCS documented by the neurosurgeon is then acceptable. When discrepancies between recorded scores exist in the chart, the score determined to be that recorded earliest in the patient's course should be entered. If there is no documentation of an actual score in the chart, then one may be calculated by the abstractor if there is sufficient information from the combined narrative nursing and physician notes to do so. No documentation of the GCS, or insufficient information to calculate it, will be indicated by entry of 99 for the GCS data element.

An example related to injury coding is also useful. In the case of a patient with a femur fracture, the most reliable diagnosis would come from an autopsy report, an analysis of x-ray films, or an operative report. Less reliable sources might be the physician's initial history and physical or progress notes, emergency department nursing record, or prehospital provider report. While physician, nursing, and prehospital provider information may give clues to the potential for the presence of certain injuries, these indications should be confirmed by more objective and substantive evidence such as the operative, radiology, or autopsy reports. Therefore, injury coding and calculation of injury severity are best reserved until retrospective chart review, after a patient has been discharged.

Finally, an example related to complications is particularly important. The term "renal failure" often appears in patient records. However in one patient this may reflect the need for dialysis, while in another it may reflect only a mild elevation in BUN or creatinine. A strict definition outlining values for each parameter considered in classifying complications (e.g., "creatinine ≥ 2.5 mg/dL requiring dialysis or hemofiltration") is essential to assure uniformity of data. Standard definitions for a number of complications have been proposed by the ACS.[1] Identification of complications is best accomplished by a designated clinician (either a trauma surgeon or trauma nurse coordinator) familiar with the exact definitions. When the arrangement is feasible, concurrent submission of identified complications to the trauma registry personnel on a daily or weekly basis for immediate entry is an optimal method of cataloguing complications.

Each data source should be evaluated to ascertain its reliability in providing a given piece of information on any given patient. Sources that are not reliable should not be routinely used to gain information. Assurance that information contained only in certain documents (e.g., ED flowsheet, operative record, autopsy report) is consistently present must be attained through education of the care providers responsible for completing these medical records.

At our institution, a resident physician intake form that is not part of the medical record is employed to facilitate acquisition of initial patient data. This form was specifically intended to contain most of the elements required for entry into the prehospital and ED registry fields. It is also possible to design such forms to conform to the flow of registry screens.

Because it is not part of the medical record, completed forms on the preceding day's patients can be submitted to the trauma registry office daily, after clinical rounds. The form itself can be easily and frequently revised without the involvement of the hospital records committee. The rates of missing forms and completeness for each element on the form are calculated and trended each month as part of the trauma service quality assurance activities. Analysis of the trends can lead to revisions to the form or educational interventions.

The residents at our institution have found the form to be helpful in making their presentations at morning rounds. The registry office has found the form quite useful in expediting the entry of initial data into the registry database and in adding to the efficiency and accuracy of data management.

Data Collection Tools

After data element selection and definitions have been addressed, it is often helpful to develop a data collection tool to aid in chart abstraction and data entry. This is particularly true in a registry that operates primarily using a retrospective chart review process. Specially configured forms will help to optimize quality by allowing for structured recording of necessary data. To ensure the greatest ease and accuracy of abstraction and entry, the flow of the tool should conform to the manner in which the patient chart is assembled, or the flow of the registry data field screens, or both when possible. Check boxes and "pick lists" that limit selections of the abstractor are often more effective than transfer of free text and narrative in maintaining accuracy and diminishing errors in data transfer. When different data are collected for more than one regulatory agency, it is most efficient to use an integrated collection tool as well as an integrated database. Duplicate abstraction, recording, and entry will consume additional resources. Reporting requirements and software considerations will often influence the decision as to whether an integrated form is feasible and single entry can be accomplished.

Data entry can also be accomplished directly from the chart into the database without an intermediate step. This practice eliminates the collection tool and mitigates errors introduced by multiple data entry steps. The retrospective chart review method, performed at a computer workstation in the registry office or medical records department, can be used to achieve direct data transfer. It is also possible, however, for registry personnel using laptop computers to enter the data directly from the patient charts while they are still housed in active patient care areas.

Most software packages will allow the user to create a download or export program and can accept an import from other databases. This may require some programming assistance from the commercial supplier of the hospital registry software or from hospital programming personnel. The capability of import and export of data reduces or eliminates the need for duplicate and manual entry. This advantage has significant implications for the efficient and cost-effective operation of the registry. Moreover, these technological strategies can decrease the time required for chart abstraction and entry, thereby potentially reducing the number of employees (or full-time equivalents) required for registry operation.

Demographic, laboratory, and financial data are generally collected by other hospital departments and entered into separate computerized data-bases. This is true even for clinical data from the ICU, operating room, and emergency department in some hospitals. These databases may be PC-based or on a mainframe. In either case, the creation of import and export programs and policies governing the electronic transfer of data elements that are common and pertinent to the trauma registry can be accomplished. This can be done in batch form on a regular basis, or even on-line in some data systems. For example, a hospital might institute a daily electronic download from the admitting office database to the trauma registry data-base of all pertinent demographic data on patients admitted to the trauma service. This would eliminate the need for manual abstraction or entry of those data elements by trauma registry staff.

Likewise, an electronic export of registry data to other external sources, such as a trauma system lead agency or the JCAHO, would eliminate the needs to use and maintain separate software and to reenter previously catalogued data. Export of trauma registry data either to other databases within the hospital or sources external to the hospital will depend on a defined case population to be transferred. This may or may not be a subset of the hospital trauma registry population. There must also be defined data set, which again may be a subset of the hospital trauma registry data set. Ideally, data elements shared between the hospital registry and the receiv-ing source will have common definitions.

The final and perhaps most important factor determining the feasibility and success of data export is the capability and willingness of the receiving agency or hospital department and its data system to accept an electronic transfer. As a result of financial constraints, the requirements for program-ming expertise and committed technical support, as well as other adminis-trative and regulatory factors, a number of trauma system lead agencies mandate the use of a single trauma registry software product by all recog-nized trauma care facilities in the system. This may be the most beneficial policy from the perspective of the lead agency. However, unless the singular software product selected has the flexibility to meet the local needs of the individual hospitals required, the strategy of using it to improve system-wide data collection and management may be counterproductive.

Such monolithic policies have contributed to the failure of individual trauma hospital registries, system registries, and trauma systems. To avoid such failures, the advantages and disadvantages of a policy mandating use of a singular software product must be considered with respect to all the contributors and users of the data. A final decision must be arrived at by consensus of all parties involved. If a decision favoring uniform use of a single software product is arrived at, the designated product should be flexible enough to meet the needs of local hospitals as well as the changing needs of the trauma system and the lead agency. This is essential, as the successful trauma system will evaluate and modify system standards over time. If it is decided to allow the use of multiple software products throughout the system, with a policy of regular transfer of a delineated trauma system data set, particular attention must be paid to the logistics and uniformity of data transfer to ensure the production of useful information.

Quality Control

The goal of registry-specific quality improvement is consistency in practice, data completeness, and data accuracy. The usefulness of the data collected by the hospital trauma registry will depend largely on the application of reliable data collection techniques and on the presence of measures that validate the integrity of the data. Useful and reliable information coming from the registry is rooted in the ability of the registry to continuously assess the data management process, identifying strengths, weaknesses, and areas for improvement. The registry must be able to act as change agent; it must be modifiable; and it must be able to reevaluate itself, as well as the changes in practice it has been used to bring about.

The process of assuring data integrity can be considered on several levels. A first level seeks to minimize interpretive errors. This can be accomplished by assigning qualified personnel to do the abstraction. Data elements requiring clinical judgment should be abstracted or identified for processing by individuals with appropriate experience.

Selective data review by the registry medical director and the registry supervisor constitutes a second level of quality assurance. During the secondary review, an independent reviewer examines each record for completeness and obvious errors. In smaller registry operations, a single reviewer/abstractor will be responsible for performing this function as a self-check on a certain number of charts. A designated physician or registry medical director may specifically review records for patients with morbidity or mortality. Quality checks related to morbidity could include the completeness and accuracy with which injuries and complications are identified. Other basic quality checks might include those related to implausible or impossible data values, such as systolic blood pressure exceeding 300 or a discharge disposition to home for a patient who has expired. Many internal validity checks may be built into registry software. Software products possessing this feature do not accept the entry of implausible/impossible values for certain data elements.

Finally, the registry supervisor should perform an item-by-item comparison of the registry input and information contained in the chart, validating accuracy of entry in a random 10% sample of cases each month.[6,7] In a system entering 1700 cases per year, this process is estimated to require 15 hours per month. Reabstraction of charts is recommended to permit continuous assessment of the quality of the data in the registry.[7] This is especially important when the registry employs more than one abstractor and/or separate data entry personnel. The number of individuals involved in abstraction and data entry is directly correlated with the integrity of the database and the degree of quality control efforts needed to maintain that integrity.

Continual evaluation of the four basic components of the trauma registry will assure the utility of the database and its ability to fulfill its mission. The four basic components are data abstraction, coding, data entry, and reports.

Data abstraction is a primary function in the operation of every trauma registry. Assessing quality in data abstraction begins with systematic, organized, and frequent reviews of inclusion criteria and the data set. The data set and inclusion criteria should be reviewed at least annually. Elements that continue to be collected as a requirement for submission to external agencies should be maintained as long as the registry continues to report to those agencies. Changes in a particular agency's required data set should also be noted and the hospital trauma registry data set revised accordingly.

Other data elements contained in the registry data set should be reevaluated for continued inclusion and changes in definition. Items that have a capture rate of less than 85% (i.e., missing >15% of the time) should be assessed with regard for their continued need to be included in the registry data set. If they are deemed to be essential to the database, the reason for their poor rate of entry must be investigated. Etiologies may rest with abstractors, care providers, or the potentially detailed and obscure nature of the missing elements themselves. Strategies to improve collection of truly essential elements may involve further education of abstractors or data contributors as to the importance of these data.

Items deemed nonessential should be eliminated. As new questions for the registry to answer arise, new elements may be added to, or substituted for, elements in the existing data set. Ongoing data set evaluation and, when necessary, revision will be required to meet the changing needs of individual hospitals and systems.

The educational background of the abstracting staff should also be reevaluated. Changes made in the method of data collection or additions of data elements requiring more clinical judgments may identify a need to change the qualifications of personnel assigned to perform the data abstraction. Some data elements, no matter how well defined, may be captured more accurately by an individual with clinical experience. Often these are items for which inadequate documentation is provided by medical staff members.[7] More accurate and complete acquisition of these elements might be accomplished by having the determination done by more clinically oriented personnel.

Injury identification and coding is a very important factor in maintaining the integrity of the patient profile. Coding standards have been set by organizations such as the Association for the Advancement of Automotive Medicine (AAAM) and the American Hospital Association. The former is responsible for the promulgation of the Abbreviated Injury Scale (AIS) and its coding format,[8] the latter is responsible for the ICD-9 CM codes.[4] A resource manual is provided by each organization. The AAAM and the American Trauma Society both offer courses in injury coding. Some institutions require coders to demonstrate proficiency or take coding courses prior to employment. There are also some initiatives to have personnel responsible for injury coding be credentialed by an appropriate national organization or credentialing body.

Coding may or may not be done by the trauma registry staff. In many institutions this function is performed by medical records personnel, a practice that may present problems with regard to the number of injuries recorded, their prioritization, and accuracy of coding. For example, some medical records departments not only limit the number of ICD-9 codes listed, they determine those that are recorded based on reimbursement considerations rather than on severity of injury or in relation to primary reasons for hospitalization. A policy allowing direct entry of these codes into the trauma registry database will necessitate an evaluation of the quality, appropriateness, and completeness of injury coding done by medical records personnel.

Some software programs exist for conversion of ICD-9 codes into AIS scores and subsequently an Injury Severity Score.[9] Use of such programs requires close attention to proper and complete cataloguing of ICD-9 codes regardless of professional background of the personnel responsible for coding or the department in which it takes place. Other software programs available allow conversion of text into AIS codes. This type of injury coding program requires an accurate entry of descriptive text by care providers and abstractors alike.

Regardless of the method used, the injury coding performed should be evaluated regularly. This may involve recoding 5 to 10% of charts as a check on reliability. In addition to assessing the accuracy of the AIS scoring and the calculation of the ISS, other coding scales used within the registry should be examined. These include the Revised Trauma Score (RTS),[10] the Glasgow Coma Scale (GCS)[11] score, and the Functional Independence Measure (FIM)[12] score. The amount of auditing required will depend on whether these scores are automatically calculated by the software or manually calculated by registry staff or care providers. Inaccurate or absent coding of the RTS or GCS may need to be addressed at several levels, such as with the prehospital providers, emergency department staff, and trauma physicians, in addition to registry personnel.

An assessment of data entry is essential to any quality control mechanism. Audits should be performed on a routine basis. Often, the software design will perform many of these functions internally. Fields or elements not regulated by internal quality control measures should be subjected to regular manual audits. Mandatory fields that cannot be left blank will require data entry personnel to enter data in such fields. Entry audits will disclose minor inconsistencies (e.g., with names: MacDonald vs. McDonald) or more blatant omissions of data. The creation of a field that identifies the individual who completed the entry will often make the personnel more accountable and aid in selecting strategies for quality assurance interventions. The entry audit can serve to determine whether data elements are missing because they were not collected during abstraction or because they were erroneously omitted during entry.

The reporting mechanism is the fourth and last component that requires review. Trauma registry data are collected and stored for one purpose, to generate reports. The lack of adequate reporting and analysis of the data may result in the failure of a registry to fulfill its mission and to be supported by the hospital. Standard and ad hoc reporting should be available. Reports created should be assessed both for relevancy and accuracy prior to their dissemination. The query process, as well as the results of the query, should be assessed. Appropriate personnel to direct and manage the reporting process should be identified. Personnel must be familiar with the software and the database to be queried. Report design will determine whether the report can be easily understood by the reader.

In summary, quality control of abstraction, coding, entry, and reporting should be a continuous process. It provides the opportunity to assess whether the objectives of the trauma registry are being met and to keep its operation relevant. As the purpose, objectives, and technology of the registry change, so should the methods of data management and registry operations.

Other Considerations

In addition to clearly defined objectives, inclusion criteria, and the existence of a quality control mechanism, several other considerations directly or indirectly affect the day-to-day workings of the trauma registry. Thus questions of staff, hardware, and software also must be addressed.

Staff

Effective operation of a hospital trauma registry requires the commitment of significant personnel and resources.[13] Typically, hospital trauma registries will require one full-time equivalent (FTE) per thousand cases entered into the registry database.[7] This estimate is to some degree influenced by the number and nature of data elements collected on each registry case. It is also influenced by the educational background of the personnel performing abstraction and/or entry and the commitments of the personnel responsible for registry operation to other trauma-related and hospital duties. Additional technical support may be required for special reports and projects, as well as for data entry.

Financial constraints may dictate the qualifications and educational background of registry personnel. The ability of the registry to use staff of different qualifications also depends on the design of the registry database, its operation, and its primary purpose. The degree to which the registry is used to provide support for the institution's program of quality assurance/improvement may exert the greatest influence on decisions regarding the number of personnel necessary and their qualifications.[7,14,15] The amount of direct involvement by medical staff, both physicians and nurses in registry operation, will also influence the amount of clinical judgment and expertise required by registry staff. The operational design of data management will also dictate whether all individuals need to be trained in chart abstraction as well as data entry. Close association between registry staff and the medical staff responsible for the daily care of patients will facilitate data abstraction by nonclinicians. It will also increase the accuracy of injury coding and the identification of complications. Having clinicians who are readily accessible to the registry staff or a part of its operation will also serve to optimize quality control and data integrity.

All registry personnel involved with abstraction and data entry should display familiarity with anatomy, medical terminology, and injury coding conventions. When the registry staff consists of more than one person, an orientation program should be designed for new registry staff, to familiarize them with the registry objectives, the database, the registry software and hardware, the data flow, and the composition of the patient record. The orientation curriculum should include tutorials on AIS scoring, ISS calculation, and ICD-9 coding, as well as other pertinent scoring tools and their calculation where appropriate. Various methods of ascertaining the total number of injuries and complications experienced by each patient should also be addressed.

Continuing education is essential to keep the trauma registry staff current with changes in the individual hospital registry as well as the field of trauma data management. Personnel should be offered the opportunity to attend pertinent classes and lectures. Educational interventions should be instituted when quality audits identify problems in data element collection, entry, or coding. The staff needs to be aware of revisions in registry inclusion criteria or data element definitions and the rationale behind them. All such revisions should be followed by an audit for compliance with new standards. Most internal educational programs should be developed and presented by the trauma registry medical director or supervisor.

Hospital trauma registry organizational schemes range from a single trauma registrar who also functions as the trauma nurse coordinator to larger departments employing several dedicated employees with various professional backgrounds and varying responsibilities in the registry office. Regardless of the number of personnel, the ultimate responsibility for registry data integrity and accuracy rests with the medical director of the trauma registry. This is usually the trauma service director. Daily operation, timely completion of chart review, and validation of data, however, are normally the responsibility of the registry supervisor/coordinator. This position is usually filled by a nurse who primarily supervises data acquisition and processing. This individual is most intimately involved with the daily routine of data management and therefore should define and modify the roles and job descriptions of the data processing personnel and any ancillary staff necessary to support registry operations.

Hardware

While trauma registries in a few small hospitals may still rely on manual recording and cataloguing of data, this type of operation has almost universally been replaced by computerized formats. Most of these are now PC-based. Computer hardware requirements are usually dictated by the software in use, the need for memory and storage of patient data, and the number of functions other than registry data management to be supported.

The actual brand of hardware used can vary with institutional preferences and budgetary constraints. Essential components of a computer system used to support the trauma registry include at least one central processing unit (CPU), random access memory (RAM), disk drives, keyboard, monitor, and printer. These may be dedicated to trauma registry purposes alone or shared between different functions and staff.

Desirable but not necessarily essential features are electrical power protection and a tape drive backup. Although the backup of data can be accomplished using diskettes, tape backup is more efficient. A modem, mainframe access, and network access capability are optional.[16]

Specifications of the hardware required to support most hospital registry software and operations include a 486 CPU rated at 66 MHz, with 16 megabytes (MB) of RAM, a 210 MB hard drive, 1.44 MB floppy disk drive, a color monitor, and a keyboard. Cost of the total system may range from $1200 to upward of $10,000 depending on a number of factors. The trend over several years has been toward the availability of increasingly sophisticated and powerful hardware at a lesser cost.

The number of workstations necessary for efficient operation will be determined by the number of registry staff members and the capability of the software to allow multiple users to perform multiple data management functions simultaneously. A file server, with specifications and speed generally determined by the registry database software, is required.

TABLE 9.1. Software considerations

Ease of entry
Reference materials (instruction manual)
Training and installation
Availability of customer service
Standard reports
Ad hoc reporting capabilities
Data display capabilities
Coding conventions and conversion features
Precalculations (e.g., transport and scene times)
Customization capabilities
Presence of internal quality checks
Access security
Cost (initial and maintenance)

Software

There are a large number of software products commercially available for trauma registry data collection and reporting. The capabilities of these software packages vary, their perceived attributes and disadvantages being institutionally dependent. No one software package can, or proposes to, meet the needs of all users. The choice of software for a particular hospital trauma registry should be made with the objectives and primary purpose of that registry in mind.

If the sole purpose is to maintain designation or accreditation as a trauma care facility, then software recommended or mandated by the appropriate regulatory agency is probably sufficient. Many trauma registry software programs have been written for use within a single hospital. Others are somewhat more generic and have focused on regional or statewide trauma system data collection. If such software is unable to collect alternative data elements or to produce the type of reports desired, however, it may not be capable of supporting other hospital-specific trauma registry functions. A trauma registry that has multiple objectives and functions will require flexibility in both data collection and data reporting. Factors to be considered in choosing trauma registry software programs are listed in Table 9.1. Costs for commercially available trauma registry software ranges from programs provided to hospitals gratis to those costing as much as $20,000. Maintenance costs generally range from $1,000 to $9,000 per year.

Reports

Trauma registry data are collected with the intent that at some point the discrete items will be transformed into useful information. This is generally accomplished through the production of trauma registry reports. The best way to assure long-term sucess of a trauma registry is to develop reporting capabilities that meet ongoing needs from the perspectives of both the hospital and the trauma system. Ideally, trauma registries should regularly produce administrative reports that contain vital information on resources, resource utilization, and finance, and these documents should become so familiar to hospital managers that the reports are deemed indispensable. Similarly, clinical information, including that on morbidity and mortality, should become so integrated with the overall quality assurance effort that clinicians feel unable to provide or evaluate trauma care optimally without them. Support for the trauma registry is broadened by involving a full spectrum of clinicians and researchers. This facilitates the development of efficient and effective programs for public information and education, injury prevention, medical research, and medical education.

Trauma registry reports can be categorized into two types: standard and ad hoc. Standard reports are built into the basic software program and can be generated automatically. Usually menu driven and be easily produced by clerical personnel, these preprogrammed reports are generally used to provide standard information to administrators and clinicians on a regular basis.

Ad hoc reports are specially prepared and require certain database interrogatory skills of the individual preparing the report. These reports are usually generated as a result of questions that arise with regard to certain trauma care issues. They are often not likely to be repeated regularly and therefore do not necessarily merit inclusion as part of the standard report software.

The number, types, and formats of both standard and ad hoc reports vary with different software products. Software also varies in its ability to modify or customize standard reports or to generate ad hoc reports. Each individual hospital must determine the priority of database query and report generation. This will influence decisions as to the software product best suited to the objectives of the hospital and of the registry. Examples of different types of report are listed in Table 9.2.

Patient log reports represent the most rudimentary of reports. The log, which provides data on the total number and identity of patients contained in the registry, is usually updated daily. At a minimum, this type of report contains the name and an identifying number for each case. The patient record report is another basic report; it includes all recorded data elements (or a select number) for an individual patient. This material is usually organized by the sequence of care and includes demographics, prehospital

TABLE 9.2. Types of registry report

Patient logs
Patient records
Administrative summaries
Activity summaries
Process summaries
Outcome summaries

care, emergency department care, surgical intervention, intensive care, complications, and discharge information.

Examples of information that may be contained in administrative summaries include patient population profiles based on variables such as injury etiology, modes of prehospital transport, time of day of admission, emergency department disposition, length of hospitalization, hospital discharge disposition, payer mix, charges, and reimbursements. Such information obviously has implications for hospital staffing, strategic planning, and cost/charge structuring.

Activity summaries provide the capability to list diagnoses and procedures by a particular trauma care service or physician. Process summaries provide information on compliance with hospital and system standards. Examples of these include reports documenting the percentage of patients who fall outside the American College of Surgeons Quality Assurance Audit Filter parameters.[1] Outcome summaries provide the basis for mortality investigations on patients falling outside the generally accepted outcome norms based on the Major Trauma Outcome Study.[2] Outcome study reports, particularly those based on the MTOS TRISS methodology, are frequently used as the foundation for quality assurance efforts.[1,2,14,15,17] These reports can be used to trend outcomes at an individual institution over time or in relation to specific interventions or changes in management strategies.

Confidentiality must be maintained throughout all phases of data collection analysis and reporting.[18] This is a crucial issue, and hospitals within jurisdictions or trauma systems that do not have executive or statutory legal protection for medical data must take special precautions to protect themselves and their patients. All data should be reported in the aggregate, to the extent possible. Data fields should be stripped of specific identifiers prior to being made available to entities outside the hospital. Finally, precautions should be taken to assure that information presented in connection with quality assurance activities is protected under that umbrella and is nondiscoverable.

Future of Hospital Trauma Registries

The success of the hospital trauma registry depends on the ability of individuals, institutions, and trauma systems to access and use the data that have been collected.

Educational programs are needed to support the growth of hospital trauma registries and trauma data information systems and to develop the personnel working in them. The development of such programs will improve efficiency, reliability, and the overall quality of the data collected.

The ability to analyze these data in a concurrent fashion for the purpose of evaluating resource consumption, cost effectiveness, and patient outcome is essential. Health care reform initiatives will increasingly require care providers to produce cost/benefit/outcome analyses. Hospital trauma registries will play a crucial role in providing these data and analyses.

Several organizations, including the American College of Surgeons, the Centers for Disease Control and Prevention, and the Health Resources Services Administration of the federal Department of Health and Human Services, are contemplating the development and administration of a national standard trauma registry data set, software product and data repository. Additionally, the Joint Commission for the Accreditation of Healthcare Organizations is developing criteria to be used in the evaluation of trauma care for its accreditation process.

With the advent of hospital-wide informatics systems, computerized records and common data collection, independent trauma registries with separate software, and dedicated staff may be replaced by a hospital data set and informatics staff. The capability of a hospital trauma registry to collect the required data, either through an independent registry or trauma subset of hospital data systems, provides essential health care information, and participates in any mandated or voluntary national trauma data management efforts is critical to the advancement of injury control. This capability can be realized only if there is a cognizance of the trauma registry's critical purpose of trauma data collection and analysis, and a commitment to allow it to serve that purpose, on the part of the hospital administration and clinical staff.

References

1. American College of Surgeons Committee on Trauma. Resources for Optimal Care of the Injured Patient: 1993. Chicago: ACS; 1993.
2. Champion HR, Copes WS, Sacco WJ, et al. The Major Trauma Outcome Study: Establishing national norms for trauma care. *J Trauma* 1990;30:1356–1365.
3. Pollack DA, McClain PW. Trauma registries—Current status and future prospects. *JAMA* 1989;262:2280–2283.
4. National Center for Health Statistics. *International Classification of Diseases*, 9th revi., clinical modification, 4th ed. Ann Arbor, MI: Practice Management Information Corporation; 1993.
5. Guyer B, Berenholz G, Galagher S. Injury surveillance using hospital discharge abstracts coded by external cause of injury (E-code). *J Trauma* 1990;30:470–473.
6. Mayer TA, Keaton BF. Data sets. *Trauma Q* 1989;5(3):17–24.
7. Shackford SR, Cooper G. Personnel. *Trauma Q* 1989;5(3):35–42.
8. Association for the Advancement of Automotive Medicine Committee on Injury Scaling. The Abbreviated Injury Scale—1990 revision. Des Plaines, IL: AAAM; 1990.
9. Baker SP, O'Neill B, Haddon W Jr, et al. The Injury Severity Score: A method for describing patients with multiple injuries and evaluating emergency care. *J Trauma* 1974;14:187–196.
10. Champion HR, Sacco WJ, Copes WS. A revision of the Trauma Score. *J Trauma* 1989;29:623–629.

11. Teasdale G, Jenett B. Assessment of coma and impaired consciousness: A practical scale. *Lancet* 1974;2:81–84.
12. Keith RA, Granger CV, Hamilton BB, et al. The functional independence measure: A new tool for rehabilitation. In: Eisenberg MG, Grzesiak RC, eds. *Advances in Clinical Rehabilitation.* New York: Springer 1987;1:6–18.
13. Pollack DA, McClain PW. Report from the 1988 Trauma Registry Workshop, including recommendations for hospital-based trauma registries. *J Trauma* 1989;20:827–834.
14. Leyendecker M, Erlich FE. Quality assurance, nurses, and physicians. *Adv Trauma* 1990;5:175–196.
15. Cooper GF, Murin P, Sheridan-McArdle M. Advances in quality assurance. *Adv Trauma* 1987;2:1–18.
16. Rasmussen ED. Computerization. *Trauma Q* 1989;5(3):43–60.
17. Boyd CR, Tolson MA, Copes WS. Evaluating trauma care: The TRISS method. *J Trauma* 1987;27:370–378.
18. Cales RH. Reports. *Trauma Q* 1989;5(3):9–16.

10
Trauma Registry Informatics: State Perspectives

WILLIAM J. SACCO AND WAYNE S. COPES

Spurred by funding from the Trauma Care Systems Planning and Development Act of 1990, many states have accelerated efforts to establish statewide trauma systems. The Health Resources and Services Administration (HRSA), implementers of the act, strongly supports data collection as a key ingredient of an effective trauma care system, stating:

In addition to the identification of the number, types, and severity of injuries, an analysis of relevant data assists in the evaluation of patient care, evaluation of trauma care standards, determination of prevention strategies, and assessment of resources needed. The availability of trauma data also serves to guide policy development.[1]

Reference 1 includes a survey of states regarding statewide trauma data collection activities. For perspective, we give a short review of the survey results. There is obviously significant variability in what constitutes a statewide trauma registry.

Twenty-two states reported having a statewide trauma registry, but only three collected data from all hospitals. The other data sources were as follows (number of states reporting each arrangement in parentheses): trauma centers only (7), some prehospital agencies, all hospitals (4), some prehospital agencies, all trauma centers (2), and some prehospital agencies, all hospitals, all rehabilitation centers (1). Five states did not provide this information.

The number of data elements collected varied by nearly an order of magnitude, ranging from 26 to 256 with a median of 100. To gauge state-perceived important purposes of trauma data, the states were asked to select among nine choices; they could select more than one. Table 10.1 gives the results for the 18 states responding.

The respondents felt the best performance measures were:

Prehospital: response and scene times; triage accuracy
Hospital: patient outcome and postinjury time of entry to definitive care
Rehabilitation: return to preinjury level, use of Functional Independence Measure (FIM).[2]

TABLE **10.1.** Perceived purposes of statewide trauma data

Purpose	Number of mentions
System quality assurance	18
Injury surveillance	16
Evaluation of patient care	15
Hospital quality assurance	14
Injury prevention and control	14
Education	14
Evaluation of hospital resource utilization and cost	13
Evaluation of system resource utilization and cost	12
Medical research	11

Thus the perceived purposes and extent of coverage of statewide trauma registries vary considerably. In this chapter we describe our philosophy of a statewide trauma system and a registry to support it, which has evolved from our experience in helping to design and manage statewide trauma centers and hospital-based trauma registries. The following topics are discussed:

Registry design
Data completeness and quality
Data process/flow
Central site management
Registry implementation
Participant feedback: Emphasis on outcome evaluations
Boldness and perseverance
Future directions

Registry Design

A trauma registry is a collection of trauma-related data in a computerized database management system. The registries discussed here store data usually abstracted from more extensive records and are not intended to be the major source of information about individual patients. We feel strongly that a statewide registry should be organized to facilitate expansion and updating, and to ensure that data can be rapidly retrieved for various uses.

As with any serious enterprise, the better the design the more likely the success. Registry designers who ignore this platitude often experience costly redesigns and financial overruns, producing results of limited value.

Data collection is a labor-intensive, costly enterprise. The data collected for a statewide trauma registry should be useful for important applications. A sobering parable follows. A March 24, 1994, *Medical Outcomes and*

Guidelines Alert article entitled "JCAHO Backs Away from Indicator Implementation Deadline" reported growing concerns over the cost and value of the outcomes-based Indicator Measurement System adopted by the Joint Commission for the Accreditation of Healthcare Organizations. In fact, JCAHO may delay mandating the program for one year (from 1996 to 1997). Many hospitals pilot-testing the 10 perioperative and obstetric indicators found that implementation was more complicated than they and JCAHO had anticipated. The American Hospital Association (AHA) and allied state associations questioned whether the indicators should *ever* be required, given the serious concerns expressed by hospitals that the data collection was too laborious and costly and that the indicators did not consistently provide information useful to hospitals.

Thus, our underlying registry philosophy is to collect only important data. As sensible as this admonition may seem, it is frequently unheeded. Many developers try to collect everything possible to collect regardless of accuracy and completeness, and end up with rarely used data items, thus draining resources that could have been better applied to the collection of the most useful items. A strategy for establishing importance, during the item selection phase, is to have a data item proponent define a report that will include the item and survey potential users to gauge its value.

We believe the chances of a successful registry are substantially enhanced by the specification of purposes and operationally defined objectives/data items that support the purposes. We believe the design process should proceed logically, in accordance with the following list; designing in this order can also eliminate superfluous data items.

Purposes. Why the data are being collected, and from which institutions and patients? These are among the questions to be addressed foremost.

Why? Selections from Table 10.1? Other?

From which agencies/institutions? Prehospital? Hospital? Trauma center? Rehabilitations? Medical examiner? All or a subset?

From which patients? All? All "seriously injured" patients? Trauma center patients? All patients who receive definitive hospital care? Other?

Feedback to data contributors. What feedback?

Future needs (change and expansion contingencies). This is an extremely important but often neglected design consideration. Registries are dynamic instruments and should be designed to accommodate new data items and methodologic changes, without costly redesigns. Audit filters, coding systems, preinjury conditions, complications, inclusion criteria, and outcome norms are examples of areas subject to change.

Each purpose should be translated into a set of operationally defined objectives. Suppose a purpose is "outcome evaluation" for all "seriously injured" patients from trauma centers. "Seriously injured patients" should be operationally defined, say, by well-defined triage criteria or specific severity score say (patients with Injury Severity Score [ISS] >12). To define "outcome evaluation," one should specify which outcomes and which evaluation methods: for example, "survival/death outcomes by the TRISS method"[3] and "median patient days in the ICU."

From well-defined objectives, it is an easy step to specify data items that support the objectives.

We illustrate the design process with our concept of an ideal state-wide trauma system, one we would want in our state. It is a system whose directors have goals of competently assessing prehospital, hospital, rehabilitation, and system trauma outcomes and care, and of serving an aggressive and courageous drive to improve outcomes and care. A statewide trauma registry should support these goals. The registry design for this concept is described next. In later sections we elaborate on other registry aspects.

A Design Strategy for an Ideal Statewide Trauma Registry

Purpose

Why? Assessment of prehospital, hospital, rehabilitation, and system trauma patient outcomes and care.

From which institutions? All prehospital providers, all hospitals, all reha-bilitation facilities, and all medical examiners.

From which trauma patients? All those who die, all intensive care unit (ICU) patients, all trauma hospital admissions for at least 72 hours from time of arrival in the emergency department (ED), and all patients trans-ferred into or out of a hospital.

Feedback to data contributors. Each participating institution would receive quarterly, semiannual, and annual reports providing data completeness summaries, system performance, outcome evaluations, and quality im-provement trends. Each institution would receive a list of its patients; seemingly anomalous outcomes, both good and poor, would be flagged for audit and for reporting back to the state.

Future needs. Anticipate such future changes as new injury coding versions and outcome norms, and be prepared to accommodate them as simply as possible.

Operationally Defined Objectives

State-of-the-art evaluations for prehospital, hospital, and rehabilitation trauma outcomes. These include PARTITION[4] (for prehospital), TRISS or ASCOT[5] (for hospital), Functional Independence Measure (FIM) transitions[6] (for rehabilitation centers), and ASCOT-NP for the system outcomes. These are described in the section entitled "Participant Feed-back: Emphasis on Outcome Evaluation."

Quality improvement and system performance measures

Prehospital: response and scene time distributions

Hospital: distributions of discharge status and FIM values for trauma survivors; number of transfers to another acute care hospital

Rehabilitation: distribution of days in rehabilitation facility

Data Items to Support the Operationally Defined Objectives

The minimal data set to support these objectives, given in Table 10.2, consists of only 38 data items. Although the emphasis is on evaluation of patient outcomes and care, the data items support all the purposes listed in Table 10.1. It is important to note, for example, that gender and race do not appear in Table 10.2, because this information is not needed for the objectives stated. Most states would want these and other demographic items for other purposes.

TABLE 10.2. A minimal set of data items to support a statewide trauma system

1.	Institution no.
2.	Case no.
3.	Age
4.	Cause of injury
5, 6.	Injury date and time
7.	Dispatch time
8.	Time of arrival at scene
9.	Time of departure from scene
10, 11.	Date and time of arrival at hospital
12–21.	Scene and ED admission respiratory rate, systolic blood pressure, eye-opening, best verbal response, best motor response
22.	Was patient intubated at scene during assessment of Revised Trauma Score (RTS)[7] components?
23.	Was patient intubated at ED admission during assessment of RTS components?
24.	Was patient therapeutically paralyzed at scene during assessment of RTS components?
25.	Was patient therapeutically paralyzed at ED admission during assessment of RTS components?
26.	Preinjury conditions
27.	Discharge status
28, 29.	Total days in ICU; total days in hospital
30.	Discharge destination
31–33.	Functional status at discharge: feeding, locomotion, expression
34.	Injury descriptions
35, 36.	Rehabilitation hospital admission values of Rasch version of FIM motor and cognition component.
37, 38.	Rehabilitation hospital discharge values of Rasch version of FIM motor and cognition components

Data Completeness and Quality

High quality data—reliable, valid, scientifically credible and defensible for the intended purposes—and submitted in a timely fashion—are prerequisites for a successful statewide trauma registry. Satisfying such requirements demands significant continuing effort. Here are some techniques that can enhance registry data completeness and quality.

1. Include only important data in the registry.
2. Develop an operations manual that contains well-defined data items and guidelines for data collection and submission, and stress that data collectors must follow the manual rigorously.
3. Emphasize to site managers and other supervisory personnel that they must lay heavy stress on adherence to the manual.
4. Provide software to data contributors that includes extensive data checks. Such checks have enhanced the quality of several national and statewide databases by identifying data items, as entered, for verification or correction. In the Pennsylvania Trauma Outcome Study registry,[7] such checks have resulted in a 90% reduction in clarification requests to hospitals.
5. Take steps to assure accurate and consistent injury coding. Inconsistent coding reduces the credibility of analyses and reports derived from a central database. Recognition of this issue motivated central site coding of injury descriptions submitted by all participants in the Major Trauma Outcome Study (MTOS)[8] and in the early years of the Pennsylvania statewide registry.
6. Provide to institutions reports on the timeliness and completeness of their data submissions (number and percentage of items completed), and comparisons with aggregated statewide values for like agencies. By highlighting institutions with good and poor compliances, these comparisons will show where improvement is needed.
7. Do on-site case reabstractions from participating institutions to determine data reliability and compliance with registry patient entry criteria.

Data Process/Flow

The concept for data process/flow presented here, which evolved from our experience in managing statewide databases, strongly reflects the computer age and our bias.

Large data providers should submit data electronically. To such providers, the state could make available tailored PC-based trauma registry versions appropriate for prehospital agencies, acute care hospitals, rehabilitation hospitals, and medical examiners' offices. Such versions can:

perform extensive checks for data quality and automatic field skips

prepare data for submission to the state

contain standard routines for generating reports on state-of-the-art outcome evaluation and quality improvement

have powerful and simple-to-use query and ad hoc report generation
capabilities

For institutions already using registries, state-provided software may serve as a consistent data checking and transfer utility that would allow users to retain their current software and satisfy state reporting require-ments without the need for double data entry; or, specifications may be provided by the state for direct submission to the central site. Thus, if the state chooses, all data submitted to the central site could be subject to the same operational definitions, data checks, and coding conventions. Such practice substantially improves the quality and consistency of the central database, greatly reduces the number of requests for data clarification from the central site, and increases the validity of studies derived from the central database.

Small data providers, which may not have resources to implement electronic submissions, should have the option of submitting paper data forms.

The central site registry should have powerful management capabilities including the ability to (1) store and process data for all institutions, (2) check for double case numbers and submission of modified data for patients whose files have been previously submitted, (3) link patient data from prehospital, hospital, and rehabilitation and medical examiner institutions, (4) allow for the backward compatibility of data as the registry data collec-tion form is updated, and (5) run standard, custom or user-defined reports on the entire database or any subset of patients. Developing user-defined reports should be an easy matter, quickly accomplished.

We stress the importance of data from medical examiner offices. These data could be linked with the central site software to provide timely and complete injury data for trauma victims who die before reaching a hospital, and to obtain more definitive injury descriptions from postmortem exami-nations of patients who die soon after hospital admission. Data from such individuals, often missing from statewide registries, are valuable for re-search and for trauma system quality improvement.

Central Site Management

The central site manager has at least four crucial responsibilities:

1. To monitor and emphasize data quality on an ongoing basis.
2. To provide timely feedback to the data submitters regarding data quality (completeness, accuracy, and timeliness).

3. To provide other feedback as specified in the registry design.
4. To cooperate with researchers and other users of the information stored in the registry.

Registry Implementation

The implementation of a statewide registry is complex. Personnel from participating institutions have to be informed of the process and trained. This section mentions several strategies that may simplify the process. An individual—rather than a board or committee—should be designated to manage the statewide registry. Also designated at each institution should be a local manager responsible for management of the institutional registry and compliance with the statewide registry policy. Operational manuals, software, and software documentation should be provided to each local manager for familiarization and practice. Start-up and periodic general information and coding and computer workshops should be held throughout the state. Ongoing activities to ensure data quality should include trauma registry update meetings and site visits by state staff members or representatives.

Participant Feedback: Emphasis on Outcome Evaluations

Medical data collection is arduous and is most often done by already overworked personnel. It is a thankless task of the highest order if data collectors and their institutions do not get feeback. Unfortunately such failures to provide feedback are too frequent in the trauma community. Registry sponsors should provide all feedback specified in the registry design. To illustrate, we give background and details for methods used to provide feedback in the ideal statewide trauma registry system outlined in an earlier section.

Prehospital Outcomes

PARTITION,[4] a method for evaluating prehospital care, is an extension of the TRISS methodology used to evaluate the survival/death outcomes of injured patients in acute care facilities. PARTITION quantitatively compares the performance of a given prehospital service to the accumulated experience of many providers used as the basis for the PARTITION "norm." PARTITION compares patient outcomes rather than such process variables as equipment, training, and adherence to standards, important as those factors are.

The key concept of PARTITION is to separate (or partition) the effects of the prehospital ministrations from those of subsequent hospital care. This division is essential, since exemplary prehospital care can be undone by poor acute care; conversely, poor prehospital care can be overcome by excellent acute care. This separation of effects is accomplished by employing survival probability estimates based on assessments of patient physiology made at the injury scene and on hospital admission and by assuming that normative outcomes result from hospital care. Therefore, PARTITION results are independent of the patient's vital status at acute care discharge.

The PARTITION norm is a logistic model whose independent variables are the patient's Injury Severity Score,[9] as determined from final diagnoses coded in the 1985 version of the Abbreviated Injury Scale (AIS-85);[10] the Revised Trauma Score (RTS),[11] as measured at the injury scene and on admission to the emergency department; and the patient's age. The model is used to estimate the increase (or decrease) in the expected number of survivors for a study group [e.g., patients treated by the prehospital service(s) being evaluated during some time period] that is attributable to prehospital care, compared to the number expected from the PARTITION norm. Significant differences (positive or negative) are assumed to be attributable to the speed and the skill with which life-threatening injuries are recognized and appropriately treated and the patient is transported to the hospital. Actual causes of differences must be determined by quality improvement reviews.

PARTITION can also be used to identify patients whose changes in vital signs from scene to ED admission differ significantly from norm values for patients who are similar in age and have similar ISS and RTS scores at the injury scene. The care provided such patients may be worthy of peer review in prehospital quality improvement programs. PARTITION has been piloted in the Hawaii and Washington statewide registries.

Acute Care

Evaluation of Survival/Death Outcomes in Acute Care

Patient survival has been the outcome of primary interest in acute care evaluations. TRISS, introduced in 1981,[3] and later ASCOT[5] have provided means for objectively evaluating acute care survival. These methods use logistic models based on patient age, injury type (blunt or penetrating), and physiologic and anatomic measures of injury severity, to estimate the likelihood of patient survival, using norms based on large data sets.[8] They can also be used to identify patients with statistically "unexpected" outcomes, worthy of peer review.[12–14]

TRISS now uses the patient's age, ISS, and RTS on ED admission to estimate survival probability. ASCOT employs the more definitive descriptions of injury in the Anatomic Profile (AP), coded valued of RTS components, and a more refined description of patient age than TRISS. For some patients, ASCOT survival probabilities are estimated not by a logistic function but by survival rates for similarly injured patients. These "set-aside" patients are those whose injuries are very serious (e.g., patients with AIS 6 injuries) or minor (those whose maximum severity is AIS 2).

Tables 10.3 to 10.8 give TRISS and ASCOT logistic function coefficients for AIS-90 based norms and the definitions of the RTS and AP components, and define ASCOT set-aside groups and associated survival probabilities and ASCOT age categories.

ASCOT is a better discriminator of survivors from nonsurvivors than TRISS, having greater sensitivities and fewer misclassifications. In addition, ASCOT satisfies the Hosmer–Lemeshow (H-L) criterion for predictive reliability for all three patient sets (adult blunt-injured patients, adult penetrating-injured patients, and pediatric patients).[15] The H-L may be the most important measure of performance for models used primarily to evaluate outcomes for patient samples rather than for individual patients.

The DEF (for **definitive**) methodology uses TRISS or ASCOT survival probabilities to compute z and W statistics to evaluate the outcomes for a patient sample. In these calculations, z measures the statistical significance of the difference between the actual and the expected severity-adjusted survival rates as determined from the TRISS or ASCOT norm being used:

$$z = \frac{A - E}{S}$$

where A and E are the actual and expected number of survivors in the sample ($E = \sum P_i$, where P_i is the survival probability for the ith patient in the sample), and S is a scale factor that accounts for statistical variation:

$$S = \left[\sum P_i (1 - P_i) \right]^{1/2}$$

Values of z exceeding 1.96 or less than −1.96 indicate significantly more or fewer survivors than would be expected from the norm.

The clinical significance of statistically significant z scores is denoted by W:

$$W = \frac{100(A - E)}{N}$$

where A and E are as defined for z and N is the number of patients in the sample being evaluated. W is the average number of additional (or fewer) survivors occurring among the sample, per 100 patients treated, than would

TABLE 10.3. AIS-90 TRISS coefficients

	Blunt	Penetrating
Constant	−0.4499	−2.5355
RTS	0.8085	0.9934
ISS	−0.0835	−0.0651
Age	−1.7430	−1.1360

TABLE 10.4. AIS-90: ASCOT logistic model coefficients

	Coefficients Injury	
Variable[a]	Blunt	Penetrating
Constant	−1.1570	−1.1350
Variables[a]		
G	0.7705	1.0626
S	0.6583	0.3638
R	0.2810	0.3332
A	−0.3002	−0.3702
B	−0.1961	−0.2053
C	−0.2086	−0.3188
Age*	−0.6355	−0.8365

[a]Where G = coded Glasgow Coma Scale, S = coded Systolic Blood Pressure, R = coded Respiratory Rate, and the G, S, & R codes are defined in Table 10.5, and Age* is defined in Table 10.8, and A = $(\Sigma AIS^2)^{1/2}$ for all the AIS detailed at row "A" in Table 10.6, and B, C, and D are likewise defined for rows B, C, & D in Table 10.6.

TABLE 10.5. Revised Trauma Score[a]

Glasgow Coma Scale	Systolic blood pressure (mmHg)	Respiratory rate (beats/min)	Coded value
13–15	>89	10–29	4
9–12	76–89	>29	3
6–8	50–75	6–9	2
4–5	1–49	1–5	1
3	0	0	0

[a]RTS = $0.9368(GCS_c) + 0.7326(SBP_c) + 0.2908(RR_c)$, where subscript c denotes coded value.

TABLE 10.6. Anatomic Profile (AP) component definitions

A   Head: AIS severity 3–5, region 1; ICD-9 CM codes: 800, 801, 803, 850, 851, 852, 853, 854, 950

      Spinal cord: AIS severity 3–5, region 1,3,4; ICD-9 CM codes: 806, 952, 953

B   Thorax: AIS severity 3–5, region 3; ICD-9 CM codes: 807, 860, 861, 862, 901, 839.61, 839.71

      Front of neck: AIS severity 3–5, region 1; ICD-9 CM codes: 874, 807.5, 807.6, 900

C   All others: AIS severity 3–5, region 1, 2, 3, 4, 5, 6

D   All others: AIS severity 1, 2, region 1, 2, 3, 4, 5, 6

TABLE 10.7. ASCOT (AIS-90) set-aside groups

Set	Description[a]	Survival probabilities (P)	
		Blunt	Penetrating
1	Patients with AIS 6 injury		
	RTS < 4	0.000	0.048
	RTS ≥ 4	0.500	0.500
2	RTS = 0, MAIS < 6	0.011	0.029
3	RTS > 0, MAIS ≤ 2		
	Age 0–54	99.9	100.0
	55–64	98.9	100.0
	65–74	96.4	100.0
	75–84	92.9	100.0
	≥85	87.5	100.0

[a] MAIS, maximum AIS.

be expected from the norm: $W = 0$ for nonsignificant z scores, since A and E are not statistically distinguishable. We believe that both z and W are required for meaningful evaluations of acute care survival.

Accounting for Preinjury Health Status

Several researchers have studied the effect of preinjury illness on trauma patient mortality. Morris et al.[16,17] studied the effect on trauma patient mortality of codes of the ninth revision of the International Classification of Diseases (ICD-9-CM) for preinjury conditions from medical discharge records, while controlling for age, and for the traumatic injury by ISS. Milzman and colleagues[18] prospectively evaluated the effect on trauma

TABLE 10.8. ASCOT patient age characterization[a]

Age*	Ages (years)
0	0–54
1	55–64
2	65–74
3	75–84
4	≥85

[a] Example: If Age* = 2, then Age (years) lies in the range 65–74 inclusive, and vice versa.

patient mortality of nine preinjury conditions, more precisely defined than the ICD items, and controlled for patient age, anatomic severity (ISS), and admission physiologic severity using the Glasgow Coma Scale (GCS). Sacco and colleagues,[19] who studied the effect on survival of each APACHE II preinjury condition, concluded that preexisting organ dysfunction has a profound effect on patient survival probability even after controlling for age, anatomic and physiologic severity, and mechanism of injury. Because of the relatively low frequency of the preexisting conditions among trauma patients, however, a strong influence of this factor on institutional z and W values was not recorded.

Accounting for Patients with Missing Data

Patients missing one or more variables are usually excluded from TRISS or ASCOT evaluations. Such patients are generally either those with relatively minor injuries, for whom the measurement of complete vital signs on ED admission was deemed unnecessary, or those who are intubated and possibly paralyzed or sedated on ED arrival, for whom one or more RTS components may not be measurable. Both sets of patients, especially those in the latter group, who are typically among the most seriously injured, should be included in outcome evaluations.

The approach we propose begins by ascribing normal physiology to patients missing one or more RTS values who are not intubated upon ED arrival. In our experience, intubated patients missing one GCS component are frequently missing all three, as well as an unassisted respiratory rate. To include such patients in outcome evaluations, a logistic function based on data from patients treated in Pennsylvania trauma centers was developed to estimate survival probability based only on patient age (as in ASCOT), AP components, type of injury (blunt or penetrating), and a variable indicating whether the patient was intubated upon ED arrival (1 = intubated, 0 = not intubated). Table 10.9 gives model coefficients for patients with blunt and penetrating injuries. The models are based on AIS-85 coding and therefore need to be updated for AIS-90. Lacking physiologic data, these models do not perform as well as TRISS or ASCOT, but they do permit the inclusion of intubated patients in outcome valuations.

Offner and coworkers also developed a TRISS-like model for estimating survival probability for intubated patients with blunt injury.[20] Their model uses the patient's systolic blood pressure and the Best Motor Response component of the GCS in place of the RTS. Injury coding was in AIS-85, and the model was based on data from patients treated only at Harborview Medical Center.

The foregoing approaches permit the inclusion of nearly all patients in outcome evaluations. The only patients excluded are those without codable injury descriptions and those whose vital status at discharge, type of injury, or age is unknown.

TABLE **10.9.** Final regression model coefficients (AIS-85)

Variable	Blunt	Penetrating
Intercept	4.7952	4.8445
A	−0.3456	−0.5589
B	−0.3270	−0.4836
C	−0.0915	−0.2601
Coded age	−0.5034	−0.4446
Intubated	−1.7081	−2.2314

System-Wide Evaluation of Survival/Death Outcome

TRISS and ASCOT also provide the means to perform a system-wide evaluation of patient survival. If we assume that a trauma system cannot prevent injury but can only treat the injured, then to minimize mortality, we would provide the patient with definive care *immediately* after injury. Such a system could be conceived as having hospital trauma care immediately after injury, before the physiologic response to injury began. The associated (and admittedly optimistic) estimate of the TRISS or ASCOT survival probability for a patient in such a model system would result from assuming that the patient's physiology at ED admission was normal. The z and W values resulting from such a "**n**ormal **p**hysiology" (NP) model would quantify the combined effects on patient survival of delayed access, prehospital care, triage and interhospital transfer, and acute care. The scores would also provide a basis for comparing a trauma system with its peers, and for evaluating the net effect on survival of interventions taken to improve system effectiveness.

Table 10.10 gives results for the usual AIS-85 ASCOT and the NP-ASCOT models for patients treated in Pennsylvania's trauma centers. With respect to the usual ASCOT norms, survival increased significantly from 1988 to 1992. The 1991 and 1992 W values suggest that for each 100 patients treated, nearly 2 more survive in Pennsylvania's trauma centers than would

TABLE **10.10.** ASCOT-based W values (1988–1992) for the Pennsylvania Trauma Outcome Study

Year	Total number of patients	W	
		ASCOT	NP-ASCOT
1988	18,130	0.81	−4.20
1989	18,220	1.19	−3.78
1990	18,651	1.36	−3.99
1991	18,892	1.95	−3.82
1992	17,681	1.83	−3.46

be predicted by the MTOS-based ASCOT norm. The trend is less dramatic for the NP-ASCOT model, despite the improvement in W from -4.20 in 1988 to -3.46 in 1992. From a system-wide perspective, these results suggest that from 3.5 to 4 more patients die per 100 patients treated than might be expected in a "model" trauma system with definitive care following immediately upon injury, despite the improvement in outcome due to trauma center care.

The results in Table 10.10 are for Pennsylvania trauma centers only. They could be used as a benchmark for comparing outcomes for trauma center patients in other states or regions. The method should be applied to all injured patients in a county or state, including nonsurvivors who never reach the hospital. Diagnoses in hospital discharge summaries might be used for such analyses, or medical examiner reports that are mapped to AIS severity scores using MacKenzie's methods. Note that the patient physiology on ED admission required for the usual TRISS or ASCOT methods, which is generally not in discharge summaries, is not required by the NP models.

The NP models are a modification of the method proposed by Sacco et al., which adopted the most optimistic estimate of survival probability ("1" or certain survival) for all patients reaching the hospital alive in order to define a Relative Outcome Score.[21]

Rehabilitation Outcomes

During the last 5 years there has been a flurry of research activity related to the prediction of discharge functional outcomes for rehabilitation patients, given the rehab patient admission functional abilities for trauma patients.[6,22–25] We believe that some of these methods are ready for use in statewide trauma registries for the assessment of rehabilitation outcomes. In particular, Heinemann and colleagues[24] demonstrate a good correlation between admission and discharge Functional Independence Measures for both traumatic brain and spinal cord patients; and Long and colleagues[6] extend the z, W "concept" to determine norms for FIM transitions in rehabilitation for brain-injured patients.

Boldness and Perseverance

The outcome measures can also be used to identify patients with anomalous outcomes, both good and poor. As mentioned previously, PARTITION can identify patients with anomalous prehospital outcomes; similarly, TRISS and ASCOT can identify patients with outliner hospital outcomes, the FIM transition models can identify patients with unusual rehabilitation outcomes, and ASCOT-NP can identify patients with unusual trauma system outcomes. Although no outcome measure is perfect, we believe such patients should qualify for review in quality improvement programs.

For the good of state citizens, we urge statewide trauma system directors to boldly and vigorously stress these reviews, despite political or participant pressures. Reports should be required from the institutions, including the following information for each designated anomalous outcome:

whether the reviewers concur with the anomaly designations, and the reasons given

actions taken to improve the good results or mitigate poor results

Anomalous outcomes may be attributed to incorrect data submissions, index failures, good or poor care, good or poor fortune, treatment delays, or errors in diagnoses, judgment, or technique.

The statewide directors should have the results trended and periodically audited to stress their importance. Institutions with consistently exemplary results should be subjected to outside audit to determine credibility. If the results are credible, the state directors should try to characterize and promulgate the reasons for success, to the level of explicit protocols if possible.

Future Directions

PARTITION Upgrade

PARTITION should be updated to incorporate the factors noted in the following paragraphs.

ISS limitations have been identified.[26] For example, patients with an ISS of 25 from head injury are substantially different from patients with the same ISS resulting from serious vessel injuries or from a fractured long bone and an abdominal injury. The Anatomic Profile describes injuries using four scores (A, B, C, and D) that more accurately describe the number, location, and severity of all a patient's injuries. The AP is used in ASCOT, a method for estimating patient survival probability, and it should be used in PARTITION as well.

The original PARTITION norm included all patients. However, as is the custom with in-hospital evaluations, distinct PARTITION norms should be developed for blunt-injured and for penetrating-injured patients.

AIS-90[27] *is now in widespread use.* Since the newer standard shows some substantial differences from AIS-85, PARTITION norms based on AIS-90 should be developed.

Time is a vital factor in prehospital care. Original PARTITION norms were based on MTOS data, obtained primarily from urban trauma centers, where times from injury to ED admission are generally less than 30 minutes. It would seem inappropriate to use essentially urban norms to evaluate rural systems, where prehospital times are characteristically longer. Therefore, we propose at a minimum to develop distinct urban and rural PARTITION norms.

The collection of necessary data and development of new PARTITION norms would substantially aid in the quantitative evaluation of prehospital care.

Offner Upgrade

Offner's method should be updated for AIS-90 and based on data from more hospitals.

Continuum of Care Trauma Outcome Evaluations

The Continuum of Care Trauma Outcome Evaluation (CC-TOE) is a model for tracking outcomes of a trauma patient from the injury scene through rehabilitation.[28] The model uses seven patient scores, two of which are based on PARTITION and ASCOT, to assess survival/death, morbidity, cognitive and functional outcomes for prehospital care, acute hospital care, and rehabilitation. Implementation of CC-TOE requires augmentation of the 38 data items in Table 10.2 with daily ICU values of four organ-specific measures and a cognitive assessment.

The Study of Non-Survival Outcomes

With the increased emphasis on care quality and cost containment, hospital resource utilization as reflected by complications, lengths of stays (LOSs) in hospital and in ICU have become increasingly important measures of trauma care quality and as a basis for reimbursement. Assessments of these factors should be made cautiously, because of the complexity of trauma patient characterization (differing mixes of injuries and ages) and variations in survival rates among institutions. For example, a trauma center may experience lower than average complication rates and LOSs because it manages younger patients, fewer severely injured patients, or more patients who die soon after injury. Another trauma center may have a better than average survival rate at the expense of larger complication rates and LOSs because more severely injured patients survive to experience longer stays and complications.

Thus, we envision much use of "matching patient" methods to compare complications and LOSs, as well as such other outcomes as hospital discharge disabilities, and percents of patients discharged to rehabilitation and skilled nursing facilities. We have used the matching method in several studies.[29,30] In those studies the outcomes for study patients were compared with those of similar ("matching") patients. The matching criteria included preinjury conditions, age, injury etiology, intubation status at ED admission, and a sophisticated characterization of injury severity.

Discussion

The United States spends 14 to 15% of its gross domestic product on health care. Concerns about rising health care costs and the large number of Americans without health insurance have resulted in many proposals for health care reform, most of which contain provisions supporting outcome evaluations as means to increase the efficiency and efficacy of health care delivery. The Major Trauma Outcome Study (MTOS), the Pennsylvania Trauma Outcome Study (PTOS), and the Uniform Data System for Medical Rehabilitation (UDSmr) are examples of large-scale outcome studies in trauma and rehabilitation that give benchmarks against which individual hospitals or systems can compare performances. The Society of Critical Care Medicine (SCCM) is embarking on a national database with similar goals, Project IMPACT.

Although trauma systems are relatively new, dating from the past two to three decades, they are extensive, covering patients from prehospital care through rehabilitation. The complexity of those systems, and of trauma patients themselves, complicates evaluations. The methods proposed here should assist trauma system evaluators by providing quantitative, objective methods and norms that can serve as a basis for comparison and go beyond the somewhat controversial preventable death studies.[34]

That the methods proposed do not constitute a complete evaluation will be apparent to all readers. For example, assessments of the triage criteria adopted, if any, and of the numbers of providers of emergency medical services (EMS), along with their geographic distribution, training, and available equipment, would all be required in a thorough evaluation of the EMS component of a trauma system. We discussed only the use of PARTITION, which compares patients treated in one system with a norm based on the accumulated experience of many providers but does not consider such other variables as resources or care process. Most other methods proposed are of the same ilk.

These methods enable evaluations of trauma system components and linkages. For example, PARTITION evaluates prehospital care; ASCOT or TRISS can be used to evaluate acute care survival outcomes, and norms are presented for FIM transitions in rehabilitation facilities. Also, ASCOT-NP provides a way of assessing by how much the survival of the system's patients differs from its goal.

Much remains to be accomplished in the realms of data collection, analysis, and interpretation. Updated norms are needed; there should be evaluations of triage and interhospital transfer in states other than Maryland; and reliable and practical methods are needed for evaluating outcomes of patients treated in nontrauma centers, where trauma registry–like data are generally not collected.

Three important data/information voids seriously limit trauma system evaluations:

1. *Data on nonsurvivors who do not reach a hospital.* There are always a certain number of patients who die at the time of injury or soon after, as well as others who die because of delayed trauma system access. Data on these nonsurvivors should be included in the ASCOT-NP evaluations of system-wide outcome.

2. *Mandatory autopsies.* Autopsy examinations provide accurate injury descriptions and severity scoring, especially for those who die soon after admission to hospital[35] and for those who did not reach the hospital. Such patients are thought to represent a high percentage of injured nonsurvivors and should be included in system evaluations. Without mandatory autopsies, they may be represented only anecdotally.

3. *Rehabilitation.* Typically, trauma registry data collection stops when patients are discharged from acute care. Patients discharged to rehabilitation should be followed so that the evaluation of that trauma system component can be accomplished.

Acute care registries could be the repositories for most of the data needed for trauma system evaluations. For the methods presented here, except those based on statewide hospital discharge summaries, required data are generally in hospital trauma registries. Perhaps the only exceptions comprise the patient's FIM values on admission to and discharge from rehabilitation, and length of stay in the after care facility. However, we believe those data could be obtained by follow-up and should be part of the trauma patient's acute care trauma registry record.

References

1. Special Report on State Trauma Data. Washington, DC: U.S. Department of Health and Human Services, Health Resources and Services Administration, Division of Trauma and Emergency Medical Systems; March 1993.
2. Hamilton BB, Granger CV, Sherwin FS, et al. A uniform national data system for medical rehabilitation. In: Fuhrer MJ, et al., eds. *Rehabilitation Outcomes: Analysis and Measurement.* Baltimore: Paul H Brookes; 1987.
3. Champion HR, Sacco WJ, Carnazzo AJ, et al. Trauma Score. *Crit Care Med* September 1981.
4. Sacco WJ, Jameson JJ, Copes WS, et al. PARTITION: A quantitative method for evaluating prehospital services for trauma patients. *Comput Biol Med* 1988;18(3).
5. Champion HR, Copes WS, Sacco WJ, et al. A new characterization of injury severity. *J Trauma* May 1990;30(6).

6. Long WB, Sacco WJ, Coombes SS, et al. Determining normative standards for functional independence measure transitions in rehabilitation. *Arch Phys Med Rehabil* 1994;75:144–148.
7. Forrester CB, McMinn DL. Anatomy of a statewide trauma registry. *Top Health Rec Manage* 1990;11(2):34–42.
8. Champion HR, Copes WS, Sacco WJ, et al. The Major Trauma Outcome Study: Establishing national norms for trauma care. *J Trauma* 1990;30(11).
9. Baker SP, O'Neill B, Haddon W Jr, et al. The Injury Severity Score: A method for describing patients with multiple injuries and evaluating emergency care. *J Trauma* 1974;14:187.
10. Association for the Advancement of Automotive Medicine. The Abbreviated Injury Scale—1985 Version. Des Plaines, IL: AAAM; 1985.
11. Champion HR, Sacco MJ, Copes WS, et al. A revision of the Trauma Score. *J Trauma* May 1989;29(5).
12. Pennsylvania Trauma Systems Foundation. Executive Summary, 1993: Annual Report of the Pennsylvania Trauma Outcome Study. PTSF: Mechanicsburg, Pa; 1993.
13. Karmy-Jones R, Copes WS, Champion HR, et al. Results of a multi-institutional outcome assessment: Results of a structured peer review of TRISS-designated unexpected outcomes. *J Trauma* 1992;32(2).
14. Gillott AR, Copes WS, Langan E, et al. TRISS unexpected survivors—A statistical phenomenon or a clinical reality? *J Trauma* 1992;33(5).
15. Hosmer DW, Lemeshow S. Goodness of fit tests for the multiple logistic regression model. *Commun Stat Theor Methods* 1980;A9(10):1043–1068.
16. Morris JA, MacKenzie EJ, Edelstein SL. The effect of preexisting conditions on mortality in trauma patients. *JAMA* 1990;263:1942.
17. Morris JA, MacKenzie EJ, Damiano AM, et al. Mortality in trauma patients: The interaction between host factors and severity. *J Trauma* 1990;30: 1476.
18. Milzman DP, Boulanger BR, Rodriguez A, et al. Pre-existing disease in trauma patients: A predictor of fate independent of age and Injury Severity Score. *J Trauma* 1992;32:236.
19. Sacco WJ, Copes WS, Bain LW, et al. Effect of preinjury illness on trauma patient survival outcome. *J Trauma* 1993;35:538.
20. Offner PJ, Jurkovich GJ, Gurney J, et al. Revision of TRISS for intubated patients. *J Trauma* 1992;32(1).
21. Sacco WJ, Copes WS, Forrester-Staz C, et al. Status of trauma patient management as measured by survival/death outcomes: Looking toward the 21st century. *J Trauma* 1994;36(3):297. Editorial.
22. Sahgal V, Heinemann AW. Recovery of function during inpatient rehabilitation for moderate traumatic brain injury. *Scand J Rehabil Med* 1989;21:71–79.
23. Heinemann AW, Sahgal V, Cichowski K, Ginsburg K, Tuel S, Betts B. Functional outcome following traumatic brain injury rehabilitation. *J Neurol Rehabil* 1990;4:27–37.
24. Heinemann AW, Linacre JM, Wright BD, et al. Prediction of rehabilitation outcomes with disability measures. *Arch Phys Med Rehabil* 1994;75:133–143.
25. Lazar R, Yarkony G, Ortolano D, et al. Prediction of functional outcome by motor capability after spinal cord injury. *Arch Phys Med Rehabil* 1989;70:819–822.

26. Copes WS, Champion HR, Sacco WJ, et al. The injury severity score revisited. *J Trauma* 1988;28(1).
27. Association for the Advancement of Automotive Medicine. The Abbreviated Injury Scale—1990 Version. Des Plaines, IL: AAAM; 1990.
28. Sacco WJ, Long WB, Copes WS, et al. Continuum of Care Trauma Outcome Evaluation. *Socio-Econ-Plann Sci* 1993;27:219–232.
29. Copes WS, Staz CF, Sacco WS, et al. American College of Surgeons audit filters: associations with patient outcome and resource utilization. *J Trauma* 1995;38:3.
30. Sacco WJ, Copes WS, Bain LW, et al. Effect of preinjury illness on trauma patient survival outcome. *J Trauma* 1993;35:4.
31. Wilson DS, McElligott J, Fielding LP. Identification of preventable trauma deaths: Confounded inquiries? *J Trauma* 1992;32(1),45–51.
32. Harviel JD, Landsman I, Greenberg A, et al. The effect of autopsies on injury severity and survival probability calculations. *J Trauma* 1989;29(6).

11
Trauma Registry Informatics: National Perspectives

Robert Rutledge and Charles L. Rice

The improvement of trauma care depends heavily on a clear and detailed understanding of the causative factors, treatments, and outcomes of injury. Effective continuous quality improvement (CQI) programs depend on concurrent monitoring of the events surrounding the care of injured patients and the results of the process. The data necessary include the circumstances surrounding the injury, the severity of the injury, the process of care, and results of treatment, including rehabilitation. Collecting, coding, scoring, and sorting this information for analysis, and reporting individual and aggregate results, are the purposes of an individual hospital's trauma registry.

To inform public policy decisions, data from individual hospitals must be centrally collected, either by region or nationally. This chapter discusses the considerations inherent in such a national registry.

Trauma as a Public Health Problem

Trauma is the most common cause of death for Americans between the ages of 1 and 44 years, and the fourth most common cause of death for all Americans. As documented in the second National Academy of Science/National Resource Accidental Death and Disability. *The Neglected Disease*, injuries are the leading cause of death and disability in children and young adults in the United States.[1] Unintentional injuries accounted for 4.6% of deaths and 19.6% of potential years of life lost before the age of 65.[2] For years of productive life lost, trauma is the most serious etiology in America, with 58 million people injured in 1989, for an overall rate of 223 injured persons per thousand population.[1] Each year, trauma accounts for 140,000 deaths, with three disabling injuries for each death. The yearly total costs of injury[2] were $177.2 billion. In addition, hospitalization charges for injury are significantly higher than the charges for hospital admission for non-injury-related causes ($12,000 vs. $5,000).

Despite its devastating human and economic impact, trauma continues to be a lower priority issue among public decision makers. Critical to any effectively targeted prevention or treatment strategy is a thorough understanding of injury. *Injury in America* calls for an adequate and ongoing injury information system.[3] Since the causes of injuries are definable and correctable, decisions about the prevention and treatment of injuries can be made only if there is adequate information about the *effectiveness* of preventive and treatment measures, as well as current and accurate data on those at risk, types of injury sustained, types of treatment, severity of the consequences, and where, when, and under what circumstances injuries occur. Such information may enable local and national agencies and hospitals to establish priorities, characterize high risk groups, target injury prevention and treatment measures within communities, and evaluate the effectiveness of injury control interventions.

Much of the morbidity and mortality of trauma is preventable. A variety of strategies have been proposed to reduce the impact of injury in the United States. These approaches include the use of several types of prevention programs, the development of trauma centers and regionalized trauma systems, and support for physician manpower committed to trauma care. Despite the desire of health care providers to improve the treatment and care of trauma patients, many trauma-related interventions are not systematically evaluated; rather, they are based on clinical experience, expertise, opinions, or expediency. Where data are available, they are inconsistently applied. Definitive information about the intervention being considered is often absent or incomplete.

A trauma registry can provide essential information about the costs and benefits of an intervention. In today's changing health care environment, consumers, payers, and policy makers demand a better understanding of the quality and the expected benefits of the services they are purchasing. Trauma registries are one vital link between the causes and outcomes of trauma and the informed development of local hospital, regional, and national interventions designed to improve the quality of trauma care.

History

The first trauma registry[4,5] and the Major Trauma Outcome Study (MTOS) were the forerunners of subsequent trauma registry systems in the United States. The MTOS was a retrospective descriptive study of injury severity and outcome coordinated through the American College of Surgeons' Committee on Trauma.[6] From 1982 through 1987, 139 North American hospitals submitted demographic, etiologic, injury severity, and outcome data for 80,544 trauma patients. Survival probability norms using the Revised Trauma Score, the Injury Severity Score, patient age, and injury mechanism were generated, and these were the inception of the TRISS methodology. Patients with unexpected outcomes were identified, and statistical comparisons of actual and expected numbers of survivors were made for each institution. The first results from MTOS provided a description of injury and outcome, as well as a method of stratification of injuried patients. These results also supported further evaluation and quality assurance activities, illustrating the value of such information and providing a springboard from which trauma registries could be launched.

Although trauma is a significant cause of death and disability in this country, as well as a major cost to the national economy, there are few population-based data available to assist health officials and policy makers in targeting resources and focusing prevention efforts.

Population

A true population-based registry would require systematic capture of all occurrences of injury, including the vast majority that are self-treated. In addition, hospital and clinic emergency departments would need to collect data on both patients admitted to hospital and those treated and released. Since the number of such patients is very large, the cost associated with the implementation of a true population-based registry would, of necessity, be considerable.

Another approach is to target injuries that are severe enough to warrant admission to hospital or to end in death in the emergency department. Although no common denominator (overall incidence of injury), will result, this approach does capture the injuries of greatest physiologic (and presumably economic) import. It is this strategy that is currently being pursued.

The advantages of a personal computer–based data system have been demonstrated by local and regional success with microcomputer trauma registries such as those in San Diego County, California, and in North Carolina and Pennsylvania. Regardless of the computer language or product used, the design of the registry, or the local, regional, or national origin of the database, it is important that there be a central repository to allow regional and national data analysis and comparison.

Data Point Selection

The success of the database is closely related to the care devoted to selecting and defining the data points to be collected. Associated with each data point are a cost and a value. Careful review and selection of each data point are critical for long-term success. The two extremes to be avoided are collecting too few data to be of any real value and attempting to collect so much information that the project fails because of time and cost constraints. Data points have been selected for the core data set of the American College of Surgeons National Trauma Registry (NATIONAL TRACS).

Coding Issues

Data must be collected and entered efficiently. In addition, because the system must allow for easy and rapid retrieval of information, it is necessary to codify the injury event, the treatment, and the outcomes. The codification used must be compatible with other coding systems to allow comparison of treatment and results with national norms. Recognized standards include the Revised Trauma Score (RTS), the codes (diagnoses, E-codes, and procedures) of the ninth revision of the International Classification of Diseases (ICD-9), and the Abbreviated Injury Scale (AIS) and Injury Severity Score (ISS) systems.

Data Set Design

A modular design that includes both a common core data set and additional data elements of interest is attractive in that it allows modification based on the changing local, regional, and national needs. The individual hospital may also want to modify the database to include additional data points. The software must be able to accommodate changes with a minimum of additional effort.

Data Validation

A design that incorporates a strategy to ensure the quality of the data is required. This strategy should include both internal validation during data entry and subsequent validation of data that cannot be checked at the time of entry. The value of the trauma registry is directly related to the validity of the data entered. Thus, a strategy for continuously monitoring data validity is crucial. Most Level I trauma centers can expect to admit between 1000 and 4000 trauma patients per year. To ensure data validity efficiently, a systematic sampling of 5 to 10% of all patients should be selected to undergo review of data quality.

File Structure

A standard format or file structure, including standardized coding and data points, is necessary for compiling and comparing data regionally or nationally. Such a standard format allows individual hospitals to participate in studies addressing local, regional, and national questions related to prevention efforts, prehospital care, immediate acute care, and long-term rehabilitation of the injured patient. In the absence of an existing national standard, the American College of Surgeons (ACS) has developed a national standard for a trauma registry patient/case definition and has identified minimal and expanded data sets. This standard was developed with national input.

Case Criteria

Recommended case criteria for inclusion in a trauma registry include an ICD-9CM diagnostic injury code between 800 and 959.9, admission to the hospital for more than 48 hours, admission to an operating room or intensive care unit, or death in the hospital emergency department. The typical trauma registry will require one full-time equivalent (FTE) employee per thousand patients admitted annually. Additional personnel may be required for technical support.[7]

Oversight and Review of the Data Set

One of the most critical features of the implementation and management of a trauma registry is the careful attention to the use of the data contained in the data set. It is of critical importance to understand the data contained in the database with respect to the inherent accuracy and biases in the data. In addition, to be effective, the data must be used: that is, analyzed, organized, assessed, and presented, so that changes in the care of injured patients can be effected. A number of locally successful registries have demonstrated that this can be done. Specific details to encourage the appropriate use of the data include the setting up of a panel of users to oversee the guidelines for data utilization.

Examples of National and Regional Registries

For any newly implemented program or intervention to be deemed "justifiable," there must be evident examples of success that can be analyzed and replicated. The following are examples of successful trauma registries at both the national and regional level.

National Pediatric Trauma Registry

The National Pediatric Trauma Registry (NPTR) is a multi-institutional database designed to compile information concerning all aspects of pediatric trauma care.[8] The registry is designed and operated to assure data accuracy and provides information to participating investigators. The growth of the database has allowed the NPTR to provide the first broad-based epidemiological description of pediatric trauma, and to develop national norms for pediatric trauma care.

The National Eye Trauma System Registry

The National Eye Trauma System Registry database is another example of a successful national registry system.[9] In a recent study, 635 work-related penetrating eye injuries were among the 2939 cases (22%) reported to the National Eye Trauma System Registry by 48 collaborating centers in 28 states and Washington, D.C. The study was of value in identifying strategies such as wider use of safety glasses and improvement in engineering controls, to prevent occupational eye injuries.

The Maine Trauma Registry

To develop a cost-effective method of injury surveillance and trauma system evaluation in a rural state, records from two major hospital trauma registries, a statewide trauma tracking study, hospital discharge abstracts, death certificates, and ambulance run reports were linked. A general-purpose database management system, programming language, and operating system were used. For each individual case identified in this way, data from all available sources were merged and imported into a standard database format. This inexpensive, population-based approach may be adaptable for other regions. The issue of linking records from multiple sources, however, needs further improvement and simplification in all such approaches.[10]

Pennsylvania Trauma Systems Foundation

The Pennsylvania Trauma Systems Foundation was created by the Commonwealth of Pennsylvania in 1984.[11] Standards for trauma center accreditation were developed. Data collected are used for quality assurance, the accreditation process, trauma prevention, and research.

North Carolina Trauma Registry

The North Carolina Trauma Registry (NCTR) is a cooperative effort among the Office of Emergency Medical Services, North Carolina's eight designated trauma center hospitals, four medical schools, the North Carolina Department of Human Resources, and the North Carolina Governor's Highway Safety Committee. The NCTR is a database system that includes records from the nine designated Level I and Level II trauma centers in North Carolina. The NCTR collects data on all patients admitted to a participating hospital for at least 24 hours, as well as all patients declared dead in the emergency department. At each hospital the data are entered via a microcomputer into a database and then uploaded to the Central Collection Agency. Data are validated on entry into the database by the trauma registrar and the physician staff at each hospital.

Data Collection

Since the injury may or may not be treated near the victim's residence or at the nearest medical facility, regional collection of injury data are highly desirable. And since injury is a national problem, national collection of data would seem to be desirable. Such national data would be useful in obtaining information about regional differences in injury occurrence or treatment and outcomes. Precedents exist in some diseases, such as cancer; but systematic concurrent collection of health-related data, other than causes of death for specific conditions, is not common.

In some states, detailed information about injury and its treatment are reported to a state agency. Although the primary purpose of these data is to identify certain injury patterns, practitioners have been concerned (with some justification) that the data are used for other purposes, perhaps with incomplete risk adjustment, possibly leading to invalid comparisons among trauma centers. This concern, valid or not, has had a profound impact on the willingness of trauma centers and trauma surgeons to participate in centralized data collection.

One solution to this problem is for a nongovernmental agency to act as the collection point and repository of centralized data. A nongovernmental agency is much less subject to Freedom of Information Act provisions and less subject to the political process. On the other hand, funding of such a project becomes more problematic.

American College of Surgeons National Trauma Registry

The American College of Surgeons has had a long involvement in trauma. Seven years after its founding in 1913, one of its first standing committees, the Committee on Fractures, was formed. That committee, now called the Committee on Trauma (COT), has played a major role in the development of institutional standards for the care of the trauma patient. In addition, the Advanced Trauma Life Support Course (ATLS®), developed by the COT, has now been taught to more than 200,000 practitioners in the US and abroad.

The Major Trauma Outcome Study, described above, was developed by the COT. Upon conclusion of the project in 1987, the COT determined that a replacement was desirable and initiated development of a national trauma registry under ACS auspices. That registry would be designed to:

assist hospitals in the collection of specific injury-related data
assist in the quality improvement programs related to trauma
provide comparative data among institutions

provide a source for national injury-related information

serve as a resource for investigators

One of the first major efforts was to determine what data points would need to be collected. Any determination of such data points would have to reflect the purpose the registry was intended to serve, as well as the cost associated with collecting the data. (With the continuously dropping price of hardware and software, the cost of *storing* the data was assumed to be negligible.) Moreover, it was assumed that some data points thought to be useful at the beginning of the project would prove not to find actual use, while new questions posed would require the addition of other data points later. Both these assumptions had a powerful effect on the design of the registry.

Another major consideration was cost of development and operation. Given the profound drop in the cost of hardware and increase in power of microcomputers, the ACS decided to base its registry on a microcomputer. This approach would allow the usage of the rich supply of existing third-party software, as well as a relatively low (compared with mainframe environments) cost of migrating to the next generation of technology.

The project is now well under way and has begun collecting data from participating trauma centers. The intent is to return to each participating institution regular reports comparing the institution's performance with that of comparable trauma centers. Another set of reports will examine the frequency and consequences of particular types of injury.

An important objective of the trauma registry is to serve the needs of investigators. To further that objective, the ACS has established a process whereby a research question can be posed, and the relevant data retrieved from the national registry. Trauma surgeons, epidemiologists, and health policy investigators are expected to use the system to address specific trauma-related issues.

Summary

Although trauma is a major public health issue, the volume of systematically collected information on frequency, severity, and outcome of trauma has been sparse. Regional and national efforts are under way to remedy this problem, and we can expect to see substantive and detailed examination of specific problems in injury control and management supported by nationally collected and validated data.

References

1. National Research Council. *Accidental Death and Disability: The Neglected Disease of Modern Society.* Washington, DC: National Academy Press; 1966.

2. Centers for Disease Control. Table V. Years of potential life lost, deaths, and death rates, by cause of death, and estimated number of physician contacts, by principal diagnosis. *MMWR* 1982;31:599.

3. *Injury in America: A Continuing Public Health Problem.* Washington, DC: National Academy Press; 1985.

4. Boyd DR, Lowe RJ, Baker RJ, Nyhus LM. Trauma registry. New computer method for multifactorial evaluation of a major health problem. *JAMA* 1973;223(4):422–428.

5. Cales RH, Bietz DS, Heilig RW Jr. The trauma registry: A method for providing regional system audit using the microcomputer. *J Trauma* 1985;25(3):181–186.

6. Champion HR, Copes WS, Sacco WJ, Larnick MM, Keast SL, Bain LW Jr, Flanagan ME, Frey CF. The Major Trauma Outcome Study: Establishing national norms for trauma care. *J Trauma* 1990;30(11):1356–1365.

7. Shackford SR, Cooper G: Personnel. *Trauma Q* 1989;5:35–42.

8. Tepas JJ 3d, Ramenofsky ML, Barlow B, Gans BM, Harris BH, DiScala C, Butler K. National Pediatric Trauma Registry. *J Pediatr Surg* 1989;24(2):156–158.

9. Dannenberg AL, Parver LM, Brechner RJ, Khoo L. Penetration eye injuries in the workplace. The National Eye Trauma System Registry. *Arch Ophthalmol* 1992;110(6):843–848.

10. Clark DE. Development of a statewide trauma registry using multiple linked sources of data. *Proc Annu Symp Comput Appl Med Care* 1993:654–658.

11. Forrester CB, McMinn DL. Anatomy of a statewide trauma registry. *Top Health Rec Manage* 1990;11(2):34–42.

Section IV

12
Trauma Informatics: Guidelines, Protocols, and Pathways

MICHAEL RHODES AND MICHAEL D. PASQUALE

There is little doubt that health care is undergoing significant change. Efforts to reduce costs and improve quality have resulted in the development of guidelines to reduce "unnecessary" variation in practice and make more effective use of health care resources. Health care regulators and payers are now requiring guidelines, protocols, and pathways for accreditation and participation in their individual plans.[1,2]

From a distance, it may appear that the successful development and application of guidelines, protocols, and pathways for trauma is straightforward. After all, trauma surgeons have ample data provided from a plethora of journals, textbooks, and newsletters. When combined with experience, this material should lead to a predictable approach for managing traumatic injuries that would result in the best outcomes. Why then are trauma surgeons and their colleagues in other fields of medicine struggling with this issue?

It turns out that "state-of-the-art" management rests in the eye of the beholder. Although a wide variety of excellent textbooks in trauma and critical care are available, most present a comprehensive and, to some extent, unbiased review of the literature, allowing the reader to choose from several options. The literature is rarely classified using a defined methodology. In addition, these textbooks may contain data that are perceived to be outdated by the time the publications go to press.[3] Journals and other periodicals focus primarily on presenting the results of a study, albeit within the context of existing literature, and usually do not methodologically classify the study. Review articles within this medium may be effective in presenting an updated perspective on select topics, but specific data classification is unusual.[4] Even on-line cybertrauma, with its enormous potential, is still in its infancy. Ironically, the abundance of information, which should be of great benefit to the practitioner, can actually be counterproductive because of the lack of uniformity of presentation, analysis, and quality.

The congressionally sponsored Agency for Health Care Policy and Research (AHCPR) began developing guidelines for clinical practice in

1989.[5] This body defined practice guidelines as systematically developed statements designed to assist practitioner and patient decisions about appropriate health care for specific clinical circumstances. The Institute of Medicine, an independent think tank providing advice to the AHCPR, suggested five major purposes of guidelines: (1) assisting clinical decision making by patients and practitioners, (2) educating individuals or groups, (3) assessing the quality of care, (4) guiding allocation of resources, and (5) reducing risks for legal liability.[6] It was believed that guidelines would be useful to a variety of groups, including patients, practitioners, purchasers of health care, legislators, and regulators. There were perceptions that health care expenditures have brought only marginal benefits, and that guidelines could help remedy the problem. Stimuli for those perceptions included a wide variation in physician practice patterns and use of services, research indicating inappropriate use of services, and uncertainty about outcomes achieved.[7–9]

The General Accounting Office reported to Congress on the experience of 27 national medical specialty societies in the development of guidelines, revealing a wide variety of methodology and effectiveness.[10] The AHCPR subsequently published 18 sets of guidelines on a variety of disease processes, mostly outside the fields of trauma and surgical critical care. These guidelines were developed at an average estimated cost of $1 million per set of guidelines. The political effect of guidelines is not inconsequential. Following publication of the AHCPR guideline on low back pain, which suggested a more limited role for spine surgery, a group of spine surgeons organized and successfully lobbied Congress to decrease the funding for AHCPR guideline development.[11] In addition, the guidelines have been criticized for being difficult to implement and for a lack of data showing effect on cost and outcome.[12,13]

Despite these criticisms, a review of 59 published evaluations of clinical guidelines meeting defined criteria for scientific rigor concluded that explicit guidelines improved clinical practice when introduced in the context of rigorous evaluation.[14] In addition, by taking advantage of techniques introduced in Canada in the late 1970s,[15] the AHCPR effort resulted in an improved methodology for data analysis. Other organizations such as the Cochran Collaboration have developed a more sophisticated attempt at guideline development by providing an electronic analytical database of the best available data.[16]

It is not yet clear whether guidelines will exacerbate or lessen litigation exposure, but initiatives such as affirmative defense and carefully designed disclaimers appear promising.[17] Excellent guideline design has the potential to reduce liability by providing immediate state-of-the-art information and by encouraging variation from the protocol, pathway, or guideline based on the surgeon's clinical judgment.[18–21]

These efforts in guideline development have taught us several lessons: (1) the process is labor-intensive and requires the brainpower of scientific organizations; (2) the implementation of guidelines is a critical and difficult step, requiring ready availability at the point of decision (e.g., at the bedside) in a time-neutral fashion; (3) guidelines should be carefully selected to impact high cost/high volume diseases, procedures, or processes. The need for integration into computerized information systems is obvious.

Terminology

A number of terms have emerged to describe the process of developing a uniform means to an end. These terms have come from different disciplines, and although they differ somewhat in scope, they are evolving specific definitions. *Practice management guidelines* are evidence-based outlines of generally accepted management approaches, which may be specific to a disease, a problem, or a process. These documents are aimed at the appropriateness of care and are best derived through national organizations and societies. *Critical pathways* and *management protocols* are bedside tools for the implementation of the nationally derived management guidelines. Critical pathways are designed to provide an overview of the entire process of care. They are primarily calendars of expected events designed to improve efficiency. They are usually specific to a diagnostic related group (DRG) or to a disease and are meant to provide a checklist for elements of care. Critical pathways have been utilized successfully for many entities, including coronary artery bypass surgery, knee replacement, hip replacement, and, to a limited extent, trauma-related care.[22,23]

Clinical management protocols, derived from evidence-based national management guidelines, are institution-specific algorithms that can be used as bedside instrument to effect care. The ideal format for graphic display of these protocols has not yet been determined. Most experience to data has been with an annotated algorithm format utilizing predetermined conventions of style. This format is thought by many to have the best bedside application and retention by users.[24,25] Several commercially developed software packages are available to facilitate this process. Ideally, these protocols are available on the bedside computer. In the interim, hard copies can be present at each bedside.

Methodology

It is impractical to expect practicing clinicians to evaluate all the relevant evidence in the literature. However, national societies or other large organizations with the brainpower and expertise can perform a systematic review (Table 12.1). This review must respect scientific principles, with particular attention to the control of biases and random errors. From these reviews, the data may be classified (Table 12.2) to allow the reviewers a

TABLE 12.1. Basic steps in guideline development

1. Define scope of guideline
2. Define major questions
3. Review and analyze data using evidence-based classification
4. Review important patient outcomes effected
5. Review benefits/risk of intervention
6. Review costs associated with guidelines
7. Invite comments from all
8. Prepare draft guidelines
9. Submit for outside review
10. Revise based on comments
11. Prepare in several formats
12. Periodically review new evidence

Source: Hoyt DB. Clinical practice guidelines. *Am J Surg* 1997;173:32–36.

means of cataloguing the power of the data. These data, when translated into evidence-based guidelines, should allow appropriate flexibility for the development of institution-specific protocols and pathways.[26,27]

Figures 12.1 and 12.2 outline scenarios for integration of guidelines, pathways, and protocols. Pathways and protocols may be applied synergistically.[28] Evidence-based guidelines using strict scientific rigor can be developed and classified by national organizations using their intrinsic resources and brainpower of investigators who now have incentive vis-à-vis the managed care imperative.[29,30] Because of the vast resources in most national

TABLE 12.2. Evidence-based classification

Evidence	Description
Class I	Prospective randomized controlled trials (PRCT)—the gold standard of clinical trials. However, some may be poorly designed, lack sufficient patient numbers, or suffer from other methodological inadequacies.
Class II	Clinical studies in which the data were collected prospectively; retrospective analyses based on clearly reliable data. Types of study so classified include observational studies, cohort studies, prevalence studies, and case control studies.
Class III	Most studies based on retrospectively collected data. Evidence used in this class indicates clinical series, databases or registries, case reviews, case reports, and expert opinion.
Technolgy assessment	The assessment of technology, such as devices for monitoring intracranial pressure, does not lend itself to classification in the format above. Thus, for technology assessment, devices were evaluated in terms of their accuracy, reliability, therapeutic potential, and cost effectiveness.

Source: Bullock R, Chestnut RM, Cliffton G, et al. *Guidelines for Management of Severe Head Injury*. New York: The Brain Trauma Foundation; 1995.

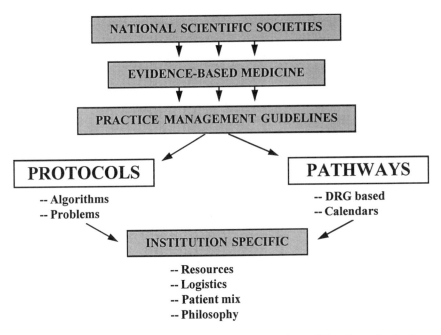

FIGURE 12.1. Scheme for translating evidence-based medicine into institution-specific bedside tools.

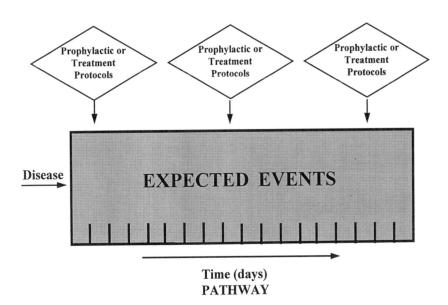

FIGURE 12.2. Pathways and protocols may be synergistic.

organizations relative to review expertise, this can be done at minimal cost compared with the expenditures of the AHCPR, which sequestered experts at significant government expense for the purposes of guideline development and analysis.

The evidence-based guidelines are then made available to institutions for the development of institution-specific critical pathways or management protocols. Using the guidelines and data classification, an institution can develop a protocol/pathway that reflects patient mix, geography, available resources, and philosophy.[1] This is essential for ultimate institutional buy-in. It also emphasizes the principle that evidence-based guidelines are available to all institutions, but that institution-specific protocols and pathways are not transferable between institutions because of the need for institutional buy-in.

The three phases of the protocol/pathway process are *development*, *implementation*, and *analysis*. Topics for protocol/pathway development are selected from the following criteria: (1) diseases, diagnoses, clinical problems, and so on that are high volume/high cost for the institution, (2) recurrent performance improvement issues in need of solution to close the quality improvement loop, and (3) areas in which nationally derived, evidence-based guidelines are available. The next step is to identify a development team with a clinical leader. The leader or "champion" must head a multidisciplinary group within the institution comprising potential users of those who would otherwise be affected by the protocol/pathway. After development of the protocol/pathway, the team presents the draft to those who will be affected in an effort to gain institutional buy-in. This effort is discussed in more detail below.

The next phase of the protocol/pathway process, implementation, is by far the most difficult phase and is guided by the following principles:

1. The protocols/pathways must be available at the bedside to all involved in the patient's care.

2. They must be time-neutral and preferably computer-based.

3. They must be preceded by a focused educational effort toward all potential users.

4. They must be strategically phased to allow interdependent protocols to come on-line simultaneously.

5. A protocol/pathway coordinator must be available daily to round with the responsible users for the purposes of troubleshooting and education. The coordinator or "protocologist" can be selected from among case managers, charge nurses, clinical specialists, nurse practitioners, physician assistants, and performance improvement personnel.

6. The bedside nurse and house staff (where applicable) are central to successful implementation.

Evaluation of the performance of the protocol is the analysis phase.[31] In many instances, incorporation of performance improvement audit filters as well as research studies into the protocols seems to be a natural fit. A guideline-derived quality evaluation process may provide a practical framework for performance improvement activities.[32] However, the temptation to use each protocol or pathway as a research study must be avoided. For the most part, protocols/pathways are not designed properly to answer research questions. In the process of trying to design them as such, the cost, time commitment, resource allocation, and ability to implement may escalate. Therefore, only selected protocols/pathways should be brought forward as research studies. This is not to say that data should not be collected as part of the analysis phase. In fact, volume, implementation glitches, points of confusion, and some generic outcome data should be collected. There should also be a commitment to revisit each protocol/pathway at regular intervals (3 to 6 months) for update and revision based on emerging evidence and institutional experience.

Initiatives in Trauma and Critical Care

Over the past 25 years, a variety of guidelines have been published on selected topics in trauma and surgical critical care. Manuals on decision-making algorithms, which serve as excellent teaching guides, have been developed.[33–35] These are primarily consensus-based and disease-oriented materials. Their bedside application has been minimal, since they are generic and are not accompanied by institutional buy-in. However, bedside-driven protocols for shock resuscitation have been shown to be superior to bedside judgment.[36] Computerized bedside-driven protocols for management of hypoxia and adult respiratory distress syndrome have also been found to be quite effective.[37,38]

In a national trauma oration, Dr. Ben Eisman suggested that as trauma surgeons, our first contract to society is to provide quality care to the injured and our second contract is to provide that care in a cost-effective manner, suggesting that we must develop guidelines for trauma care.[39] The concept of protocols for trauma management is certainly not new. Over 25 years ago, Champion and his colleagues (then at the Shock Trauma Center in Baltimore) developed protocols for trauma care, many of which have evolved into the current Advanced Trauma Life Support (ATLS™) guidelines. Other prominent surgeons have published examples of decision trees for specific injury in trauma-related diseases, and literally hundreds of immediate management algorithms for injury care have appeared in the literature. Many of these are institution-specific and are limited to initial resuscitation or surgical management. Although clinically important, they may not affect the major cost of trauma management.

The American College of Surgeons (ACS) has published guidelines for triage of the injured patient as well as guidelines designed for the first hour of trauma resuscitation.[40,41] These latter guidelines, known as the Advanced

TABLE 12.3. Description of the power of the data

Standards	Represent accepted principles of patient management that reflect a high degree of clinical certainty (usually data from class I, Table 12.2)
Guidelines	Represent a particular strategy or range of management strategies that reflect a moderate clinical certainty (usually class II data)
Options	Are there remaining strategies for patient management for which there is unclear clinical certainty (usually class III data)

Source: Bullock R, Chestnut RM, Clifton G, et al. *Guidelines for Management of Severe Head Injury*. New York: The Brain Trauma Foundation; 1995.

Trauma Life Support Course, exemplify a process incorporating recurrent analysis of the effectiveness and application of the materials. The ACS guidelines have been modified five times through both evidence-based and consensus-based mechanisms. More recently, the Brain Trauma Foundation has published evidence-based guidelines on 13 areas of head injury management.[42] These guidelines were developed through rigorous scientific analysis and subsequent classification of the data. Table 12.2 outlines the classification system utilized. Based on the data classification, recommendations (standards, guidelines, or options: Table 12.3) were made in the 13 specified areas. These recommendations can be utilized to develop a protocol for acute head injury management that can be applied at the bedside.

The Society for Critical Care Medicine has published guidelines on analgesia/sedation and neuromuscular blockade.[43,44] Guidelines for fever workup are currently under development. The Eastern Association for the Surgery of Trauma has developed evidence-based guidelines for deep venous thrombosis (DVT) prophylaxis, management of colon injury, radiologic cervical spine clearance, and evaluation of blunt cardiac injury. These evidence-based guidelines will be distributed for subsequent institution-specific incorporation using the methodologies described in this chapter.

Gaining Institutional Buy-In

Most physicians are skeptical of guidelines, protocols, and pathways. The perception of "cookbook" care is counterintuitive to the principles of surgical training, especially for surgeons trained more than 15 years ago. However, surgeons are constantly searching for evidence to guide them in patient care matters. This pursuit can be very frustrating in view of the plethora of informational sources of varying consistency and quality. Nursing personnel and technicians are not immune from guideline skepticism; however, their basic training is more aligned to the protocol concept. Their "buy-in" to the guideline/protocol/pathway concept is as important, and in some instances more important, than that of the physicians'.

The keys to institutional buy-in are inclusion and education.[1,45] The availability of nationally derived, evidence-based guidelines can set the stage for educating the potential users of a protocol or pathway. The presentation of the guidelines should be structured and interactive, such that an institutional committee of the potential users of a protocol or pathway to be developed can work to create an institution-specific protocol or pathway. Once the protocol or pathway has been developed, it may be presented to the potential users in a conference format. Algorithms are useful formats for protocols, whereas care maps are helpful formats for pathways. The presentation must emphasize where the recommendations are based on class I data (standards), class II data (guidelines), or class III data (options). It must be clear that the protocol/pathway is not rigid and, in fact, is expected to change. A mandatory review cycle of every 6 to 12 months facilitates that process.

A useful technique in consensus building among the potential users, known as the "modified consensus rule," allows the protocol to move forward if the simple majority of users agree to *try it, even though they may not entirely agree with it*. This allows for reservations to be expressed in a nonconfrontational fashion. Each protocol/pathway must contain a disclaimer stating that variation from the protocol is not only acceptable but is expected when the clinician decides that variation is in the best interest of the patient.

Another important issue in institutional buy-in is the conference format in which the protocols/pathways are presented. It is essential that the users meet periodically to allow educational exchange to occur. Fortunately for trauma and surgical critical care clinicians, such conferences are already part of most departmental structures. This educational effort is rarely successful when attempted through ad hoc committees involving multiple departments that are not scheduled to meet on a regular basis. Gaining an institutional buy-in of the protocol/pathway requires persistence and patience.

The next area of buy-in occurs in the implementation stage. Protocols/pathways will work if they are immediately available to physicians and nurses in a time-neutral fashion when decisions must be made. As mentioned previously, a "protocologist" in the person of a case manager, clinical specialist, trauma coordinator, physician assistant, nurse practitioner, or performance improvement coordinator is essential to success. Constant attention to potential glitches is imperative. Educational conferences such as grand rounds and nursing in-services should be focused around the topics of the protocols when the opportunity presents. The development of protocol is frequently the end result of a performance improvement project undertaken in response to obligations imposed on trauma and surgical critical care programs by outside forces. Meeting a majority of the performance improvement objectives, as well as some of the educational and research objectives of the institution and the training program, can be a more efficient use of energy and thereby provide an incentive to the users.

Attention to format cannot be overemphasized in gaining institutional buy-in. If protocols, algorithms, or care maps are to be in hard copy, they must be aesthetic, user-friendly, and functional. Constant attention must be paid to improving clarity and access at the bedside. Ultimately, incorporation into computer-based bedside decision analysis will greatly facilitate this process.

Although pride in the guideline/protocol/pathway development process is helpful, an institution must guard against individual or institutional ownership of a protocol. Such attitudes may emerge insidiously because of the enormous energy expended in development and implementation. The ability to change and share should be recognized and rewarded. In some instances, patients or patients' families can participate in the protocol or pathway. Educating the family about the expectations as well as the probability of exceptions can be very rewarding in gaining provider/patient/family rapport.

Institutional buy-in is neither easy nor permanent. It requires a commitment to education through evidence-based medicine that is available at the bedside in a time-neutral fashion to the provider team. It is useful to begin the process with one or two protocols to gain experience with the process. Although high volume/high impact issues are the primary targets of protocols/pathways, initiatives should begin with some of the less complex protocols/pathways—for example, DVT prophylaxis, stress ulcer prophylaxis, treatment of cerebral concussion, and screening for blunt myocardial injury.

Examples

Ideally, protocols and pathways should be developed from nationally derived, evidence-based guidelines. These protocols and pathways should be institution-specific to recognize resources, geography, patient mix, and philosophy. In trauma and surgical critical care, there are only a few examples of nationally derived, evidence-based guidelines; however, many are currently under development. The following examples of guidelines, protocols, and pathways are from a variety of sources. Institution-specific pathways and protocols that have not had the benefit of nationally derived, evidence-based guidelines can work, but their development is a much more labor-intensive process, and the resulting products lack the power of nationally derived guidelines for institutional buy-in.

Nationally Derived, Evidence-Based Guidelines

Optimal Resources for Care of the Injured Patient[40]

1. *Source.* American College of Surgeons Committee on Trauma.
2. *Methodology.* Primarily consensus-based, with mandatory periodic revisions, moving toward an evidence-based approach with classification of data.
3. *Utility.* Provides the framework for trauma center development and verification.

Advanced Trauma Life Support[41]

1. *Source.* American College of Surgeons Committee on Trauma.
2. *Methodology.* Consensus-based, mandatory periodic review, moving toward evidence-based approach with classification of data.
3. *Utility.* Provides a platform for the first hour of care of the acutely injured patient; primarily designed for the non–trauma center environment but is used as a resource for many institution-specific protocols in trauma centers. This national guideline, although primarily derived through consensus-based rather than evidence-based medicine, has had an enormous impact both nationally and internationally on unifying the approach for the first hour of care of the acutely injured. It is, by far, the best example of the power of an educational focus as the means of implementation.

Management of Acute Head Injury[46]

1. *Source.* Brain Trauma Foundation.
2. *Methodology.* Evidence-based through extensive literature review and data classification.
3. *Utility.* Thirteen areas of head injury management were critically reviewed with the development of standards, guidelines, and options.
4. An institution-specific protocol based on these guidelines was developed by the users (neurosurgeons, trauma surgeons, neurosurgical ICU nurses, and respiratory technicians). The protocol in Figure 12.3 reflects an institution-specific philosophy, patient mix, geography, and resources. Albumin use for reexpansion, which has been shown to be beneficial in spontaneous subarachnoid hemorrhage but not in traumatic brain injury, was incorporated into the protocol, reflecting a philosophy of the neurosurgeons involved in utilizing this protocol. This change demonstrates recognition of the lack of evidence supporting the value of albumin volume expansion in head injuries. It also serves as a reminder that evidence-based medicine will provide the best available data, but in real life, only a small fraction of these data will be class I. The majority of decisions will be based on class II and class III data.

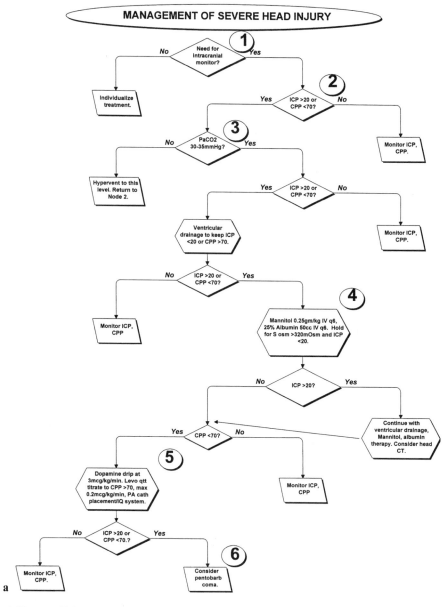

FIGURE 12.3. An institution-specific protocol for management of severe head injury at the Lehigh Valley Hospital based on guidelines developed by the Brain Trauma Foundation: (a) flowsheet and (b) key.

Agitation Sedation in the Intensive Care Unit[43]

1. *Source.* Society of Critical Care Medicine.

2. *Methodology.* Evidence-based through extensive literature review and data classification.

3. *Utility.* Provides a platform for the use of analgesic, sedative, and neuroleptic agents in the intensive care unit. Protocols may be developed from this to deal with performance improvement issues such as self-extubation, inadvertent tube removal, and barotrauma.

MANAGEMENT OF SEVERE HEAD INJURY

(1) ICP monitoring should be considered in patients with a GCS of ≤8 on admission as well as a positive CT finding (intracranial hematoma, contusion, edema, or compressed cisterns). If a patient had a GCS ≤8 with what was considered to be a relatively normal CT scan, they should be considered for monitoring only if they meet two of the following criteria:
- Age >40 years
- Unilateral or bilateral motor posturing
- SBP ≤90 that is refractory to appropriate volume therapy (Option)

(2) Maintenance of a CPP >70mmHg is a therapeutic option which may be associated with substantial reduction in mortality and improvement in quality survival. It is likely to enhance perfusion to ischemic regions of the brain following severe traumatic brain injury (Option). ICP treatment should be initiated at an upper threshold of 20-25mmHg (Guideline).

(3) Hyperventilation may be necessary for brief periods when there is acute neurologic deterioration or for longer periods if there is intracranial hypertension refractory to sedation, paralysis, CSF drainage, and osmotic diuretics.

(4) Hypovolemia should be avoided and monitoring with a foley catheter as well as some measure of central venous pressure is recommended. Serum osmolarity should be kept below 320 because of a concern for renal failure (Guideline).

(5) If after attempting to control ICP the cerebral perfusion pressure remains below 70, renal dose Dopamine should be started and a Levophed drip should be titrated to elevate the mean arterial pressure such that the CPP can be maintained above 70mmHg. Assessment of cardiac index needs to be instituted. This may either be by placement of a pulmonary arterial catheter or by utilization of the IQ System.

(6) If, after the above measures, CPP still cannot be maintained above 70mmHg, Pentobarb coma should be considered and notification of Neurosurgery should be done. Pentobarb coma protocol includes a 10mg/kg bolus over 30 minutes followed by 5mg/kg every hour for three hours. This is followed by 1mg/kg/hr maintenance dose so that the serum level is in the range of 3-4mg% and adjusted for burst suppression pattern and/or ICP control.

Recommendations by the Brain Trauma Foundation include trying to achieve full nutritional replacement by the seventh day, preferably by the enteral route. Our policy is to try to achieve enteral feedings as soon possible. Seizure prophylaxis needs to be decided upon on an individual basis.

b

FIGURE 12.3. *Continued*

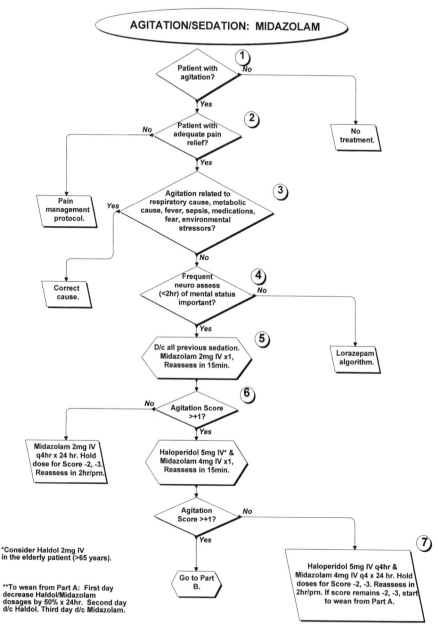

Figure 12.4. Institution-specific protocol for management of agitation/sedation with Midazolam based on evidence-based guidelines developed by the Society of Critical Care Medicine: (a–c) flowsheet and (d) key.

4. An institution-specific protocol based on the nationally derived guidelines and reflecting the resources, geography, patient mix, and philosophy is outlined in Figure 12.4.

Prevention of Intravascular-Device-Related Infections[47]

1. *Source.* Hospital Infection Control Practices Advisory Committee, Centers for Disease Control and Prevention.
2. *Methodology.* Evidence-based through extensive literature review and data classification.

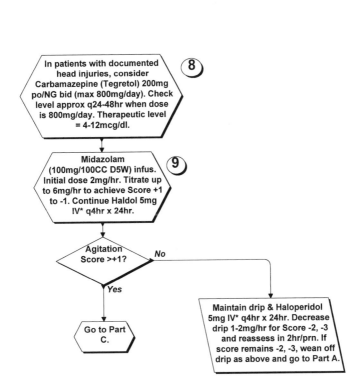

AGITATION/SEDATION: MIDAZOLAM

In patients with documented head injuries, consider Carbamazepine (Tegretol) 200mg po/NG bid (max 800mg/day). Check level approx q24-48hr when dose is 800mg/day. Therapeutic level = 4-12mcg/dl. ⑧

Midazolam (100mg/100CC D5W) infus. Initial dose 2mg/hr. Titrate up to 6mg/hr to achieve Score +1 to -1. Continue Haldol 5mg IV* q4hr x 24hr. ⑨

Agitation Score >+1?   No

Yes

Go to Part C.

Maintain drip & Haloperidol 5mg IV* q4hr x 24hr. Decrease drip 1-2mg/hr for Score -2, -3 and reassess in 2hr/prn. If score remains -2, -3, wean off drip as above and go to Part A.

*Consider Haldol 2mg in the elderly patient (>65 yrs).

To wean from Part B: first day, decrease Midazolam drip 1-2mg/hr until off and go to Part A Node 7.   **b

FIGURE 12.4. *Continued*

3. *Utility*. Provides guidelines for the use and care of peripheral arterial and venous catheters, central venous and arterial catheters, peripherally inserted central venous catheters, and pressure-monitoring systems.

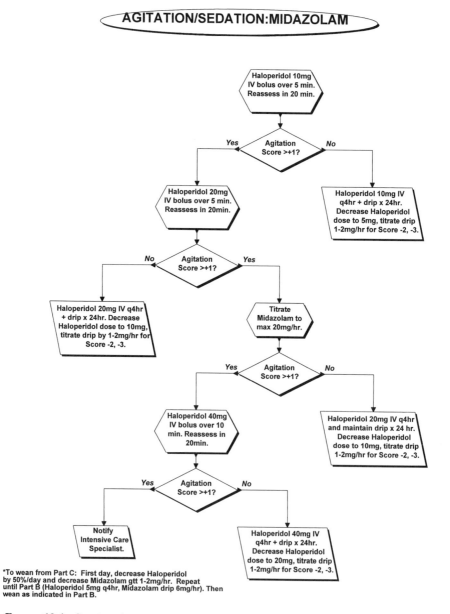

AGITATION/SEDATION:MIDAZOLAM

Haloperidol 10mg IV bolus over 5 min. Reassess in 20 min.

Agitation Score >+1?

Yes → Haloperidol 20mg IV bolus over 5 min. Reassess in 20min.

No → Haloperidol 10mg IV q4hr + drip x 24hr. Decrease Haloperidol dose to 5mg, titrate drip 1-2mg/hr for Score -2, -3.

Agitation Score >+1?

No → Haloperidol 20mg IV q4hr + drip x 24hr. Decrease Haloperidol dose to 10mg, titrate drip by 1-2mg/hr for Score -2, -3.

Yes → Titrate Midazolam to max 20mg/hr.

Agitation Score >+1?

Yes → Haloperidol 40mg IV bolus over 10 min. Reassess in 20min.

No → Haloperidol 20mg IV q4hr and maintain drip x 24 hr. Decrease Haloperidol dose to 10mg, titrate drip 1-2mg/hr for Score -2, -3.

Agitation Score >+1?

Yes → Notify Intensive Care Specialist.

No → Haloperidol 40mg IV q4hr + drip x 24hr. Decrease Haloperidol dose to 20mg, titrate drip 1-2mg/hr for Score -2, -3.

*To wean from Part C: First day, decrease Haloperidol by 50%/day and decrease Midazolam gtt 1-2mg/hr. Repeat until Part B (Haloperidol 5mg q4hr, Midazolam drip 6mg/hr). Then wean as indicated in Part B.

c

FIGURE 12.4. *Continued*

AGITATION/SEDATION: MIDAZOLAM

(1) Agitation is defined as excessive motor activity which is usually nonpurposeful and associated with internal tension. It usually interferes with patient care or clearly requires physical or chemical restraints to prevent damage to persons or property.

(2) Pain is an obvious and frequent source of discomfort which can lead to agitation. Often pain is undertreated, therefore every effort should be made to assess for adequate analgesia and relief.

(3) The underlying physiological cause of agitation should always be considered prior to initiation of the protocol as well as with each medication administered. Respiratory causes are considered to be hypoxia, anoxia, or hypercapnea. Metabolic related causes are considered to be DTs, encephalopathies, hypoglycemia, and hyponatremia. Environmental causes are considered to be sleep deprivation, excess noise, and sensory overload.

(4) If frequent neurologic assessment (<2hr) is deemed important, Midazolam (Versed[R]) is the more appropriate choice. If short-term sedation is desired, Propofol may also be considered. Propofol, a nonopoid, has a short duration of action that allows rapid awakening for assessment, examination, and extubation.

If it is felt that the patient will require sedation for a prolonged period of time, i.e. >5 days, consideration should be given to go off protocol in favor of longer acting agents, i.e. Diazepam (Valium[R]).

(5) As the protocol is initiated, all previous sedation orders (ie. Diazepam, Lorazepam, or Midazolam) will be discontinued. This does not include analgesia (ie. Morphine, Fentanyl).

(6) Agitation will be measured using a modified version of the Ramsay Scale. A target score of +1 to -1 is desired. The patient's level of agitation should be assessed and scored each time a medication is given/prn. The score and the administered medications must then be documented on the Medication Administration Record (MAR).

(7) This node will be considered an entry point for weaning from Part B.

(8) Carbamezepine, an anticonvulsant, has been shown to effectively manage agitation in the head-injured patient. Head injury ranges from concussion to coma.

Do not increase dose if adequately controlled on 800mg/day even if level is subtherapeutic.

If level is >12mcg/dl, decrease dose by 200mg/day and recheck level in approx 48hrs after dose change.

Wean drug off slowly due to risk of seizures secondary to abrupt withdrawal.

(9) Additional PRN doses of benzodiazepines and Haloperidol may be needed until the drip is available from pharmacy. Discontinue PRN doses after drip is titrated to effect.

AGITATION-SEDATION SCALE RECORD

Score	Description	Example
+3	Immed threat to safety	Pulling at endotracheal tube or catheters, trying to climb over bedrail, striking at staff
+2	Dangerously agitated	Requiring physical restraints and frequent verbal reminding of limits. biting endotracheal tube. thrashing side to side.
+1	Agitated	Physically agitated, attempting to sit up, calms down to verbal instructions
0	Calm and cooperative	Calm, arousable, follows commands
-1	Oversedated	Difficult to arouse or unable to attend to conversation or commands
-2	Very oversedated	Awakens to noxious stimuli only
-3	Unarousable	Does not awaken to any stimuli

d

FIGURE 12.4. *Continued*

Perioperative Cardiovascular Evaluation for Noncardiac Surgery[48]

1. *Source.* American College of Cardiology/American Heart Association Task Force on Practice Guidelines.
2. *Methodology.* Extensive data review without formal classification. The data are weighted by expert panels and algorithms are developed.

3. *Utility*. Guidelines are developed for anesthetic considerations, perioperative surveillance, postoperative therapy and long-term management, general approach to the patient, disease-specific approaches, and cost implications.

Summary

The development of guidelines, protocols, and pathways for trauma is part of a national effort in medicine to control cost and improve quality of care by reducing unnecessary practice variation. It is imperative that the two go hand in hand and that the focus always be on improving the quality of care. If done properly, guidelines will ensure accomplishment of these goals and, at the same time, will be cost-effective. The methodologies and initiatives are evolving rapidly.

Defining the terminology and understanding the methodology are essential. Nationally derived, evidence-based guidelines using existing scientific organizations and vigorous scientific methods can be used to develop institution-specific guidelines, protocols, and pathways reflecting local resources, case mix, geography, and philosophy. Local modification, implementation, and analysis must be centered on institutional buy-in, focused education, and incorporation into time-neutral and convenient bedside tools as part of information management technology.

References

1. Wise CG, Billi JE. A model for practice guideline adaptation and implementation: Empowerment of the physician. *J Commission J Qual Improvement* 1995;21:465–476.
2. Woolf SH. Practice guidelines, a new reality in medicine: Methods of developing guidelines. *Arch Intern Med* 1992;152:946.
3. Antman EM, Lau J, Kupelnick B, et al. A comparison of results of meta-analyses of randomized control trials and recommendations of clinical experts: Treatment of myocardial infarction. *JAMA* 1992;268:240–248.
4. Cook DJ, Witt LG, Cook RJ, Guyatt GH. Stress ulcer prophylaxis in the critically ill: A meta-analysis. *Am J Med* 1991;91:519–527.
5. Agency for Health Care Policy and Research. *Interim Manual for Clinical Practice Guideline Development*. Rockville, MD: AHCPR; May 1991.
6. Institute of Medicine. *Guidelines for Clinical Practice: From Development to Use*. Washington, DC: National Academy Press; 1992.
7. Detsky AS. Regional variation in medical care. *N Engl J Med* 1995;333:589–590.
8. Blumenthal D. The variation phenomenon in 1994. *N Engl J Med* 1994;331: 1017–1018.
9. Leape LL. Error in medicine. *JAMA* 1994;272:1851–1857.
10. U.S. General Accounting Office. Report to Congressional Requesters. Practice Guidelines: The Experience of the Medical Specialty Societies. Washington, DC: U.S. GAO; 1991.

11. Rodrigue G. Death of health agency raises questions of Congress' judgment. *Dallas Morning News*, Sept 3, 1995.

12. Kangilaski J. Physicians are slow to update treatment plan options. *American Medical News*, Jan 15, 1996, p 4.

13. Prager LO. Obstacles seen in physician use of guidelines. *American Medical News*, Feb 19, 1996, p 3.

14. Grimshaw JM, Russell IT. Effect of clinical guidelines on medical practice: A systematic review of rigorous evaluations. *Lancet* 1993;342:1317–1322.

15. Canadian Task Force on the Periodic Health Examination. The periodic health examination. *Can Med Assoc J* 1979;121:1193–1254.

16. Bero L, Rennie D. The Cochrane Collaboration: Preparing, maintaining, and disseminating systematic reviews of the effects of health care. *JAMA* 1995;274:1935–1938.

17. The Maine Experiment. *Bull Am Coll Surg* 1994, 1995.

18. Hyams AL, Brandenbury JA, Lipsitz SR, et al. Practice guidelines and malpractice litigation: A two-way street. *Ann Intern Med* 1995;122:450–455.

19. Ayres JD. The use and abuse of medical practice guidelines. *J Legal Med* 1994;15:421–443.

20. Ferrara K, Mitchell S, Price C, et al. *Legal Issues Associated with the Use and Development of Practice Guidelines.* Oak Brook, IL, UHC Services Corp; 1995.

21. Jutras D. Clinical practice guidelines as legal norms. *Can Med Assoc J* 1993;148:905–908.

22. A critical pathway in trauma. *Traumagram* Winter 1995/1996;20:5,9,10.

23. Latini EE, Foote W. Obtaining consistent quality patient care for the trauma patient by using a critical pathway. *Crit Care Nurs Q* 1992;15:51.

24. Hadorn DC, McCormick K, Diokno A. An annotated algorithm approach to clinical guideline development. *JAMA* 1992;267:3311.

25. Neale EJ, Chang AMZ. Clinical algorithms. *Med Teacher* 1991;13:317.

26. Cook DJ, Sibbald WJ, Vincent J-L, Cerra FB, Evidence Based Medicine in Critical Care Group. Evidence based critical care medicine: What is it and what can it do for us? *Crit Care Med* 1996;24:334–337.

27. Guyatt GH, Sackett DJ, Sinclair JC, et al. Users' guides to the medical literature. IX. A method for grading health care recommendations. Evidence-Based Medicine Working Group. *JAMA* 1995;274:1800–1804.

28. Schriefer J. The synergy of pathways and algorithms: Two tools work better than one. *Jt Commission J Qual Improvement* 1994;20:485–499.

29. Lewis S. Paradox, process and perception: The role of organizations in clinical practice guidelines development. *Can Med Assoc J* 1995;153:1073–1077.

30. Brown JB, Shye D, McFarland B. The paradox of guideline implementation: How AHCPR's depression guideline was adapted at Kaiser Permanente Northwest Region. *J Commission J Qua Improvement* 1995;21:5–21.

31. Basinski ASH. Evaluation of clinical practice guidelines. *Can Med Assoc J* 1995;153:1575–1581.

32. Schoenbaum SC, Sundwall DN, Bergman D, et al. *Using Clinical Practice Guidelines to Evaluate Quality of Care*, vol. 1 and 2, AHCPR 95-0045. Rockville, MD: Agency for Health Care Policy and Research; 1995.

33. Moore EE, Eiseman B, Van Way CW. *Critical Decisions in Trauma.* St Louis: CV Mosby; 1984.

34. Demling RH, Wilson RF. *Decision Making in Surgical Critical Care.* Philadelphia: BC Decker; 1988.
35. Don H. *Decision Making in Critical Care.* Philadelphia: BC Decker; 1985.
36. Shoemaker WC, Hopkins JA. Clinical aspects of resuscitation with and without an algorithm: Relative importance of various decisions. *Crit Care Med* 1983;11:630.
37. Morris AH. Protocol management of adult respiratory distress syndrome. *New Horiz* 1993;1:593–602.
38. Reed RL, Sladen RN. An algorithm for hypoxia management. *Trauma Q* 1994;11:4–17.
39. Eiseman B. Our second responsibility in trauma care: A new clause in the social contract. *Bull Am Coll Surg* 1994(March);79:23.
40. American College of Surgeons Committee on Trauma. *Resources for Optimal Care of the Injured Patient: 1997.* Chicago: American College of Surgeons; 1997.
41. American College of Surgeons Committee on Trauma. *Advanced Trauma Life Support Program for Physicians.* Chicago: American College of Surgeons; 1997.
42. Hoff JT. Special book review and synopsis: *Guidelines for Management of Severe Head Injury. J Trauma* 1996;39:1048–1050.
43. Shapiro BA, Warren J, Egol AB, et al. Practice parameters for intravenous analgesia and sedation for adult patients in the intensive care unit: An executive summary. *Crit Care Med* 1995;23:1596–1600.
44. Shapiro BA, Warren J, Egol AB, et al. Practice parameters for sustained neuromuscular blockade in the adult critically ill patient: An executive summary. *Crit Care Med* 1995;23:1601–1605.
45. Rhodes M. Practice management guidelines for trauma care. Presidential address, Seventh Scientific Assembly of the Eastern Association for the Surgery of Trauma. *J Trauma* 1994;37:635.
46. Bullock R, Chestnut RM, Clifton G, et al. *Guidelines for the Management of Severe Head Injury.* The Brain Trauma Foundation; 1995.
47. Pearson ML, Hospital Infection Control Practices Advisory Committee. Guideline for prevention of intravascular device-related infections. *Infect Control Hosp Epidemiol* 1996;17:438–471.
48. Eagle KA, ACC/AHA Task Force. Guidelines for perioperative cardiovascular evaluation for noncardiac surgery. Report of the American College of Cardiology/American Heart Association Task Force on Practice Guidelines (Committee on Perioperative Cardiovascular Evaluation for Noncardiac Surgery). *J Am Coll Cardiol* 1996;27:910–948.

Index

261